Routledge Revivals

Team Care in General Practice

When this book was originally published in 1976, general practice had developed enormously in the preceding years and one of the most important changes was the creation of the Primary Health Care Team. This book provides the context for how the 'new-style' general practice came about and examines the Primary Health Care Team in action. Part 1 discusses the rapid development of general practice in Britain. It selects one Primary Health Care Team and describes a detailed workload audit carried out in 1972. One of the most significant findings was the comparatively small workload for the General Practitioner when they were integrated into a well-functioning team. Part 2 analyses the results of a detailed Patient Satisfaction Survey, conducted by a university sociology team. Several hypotheses were tested, all relating to the satisfaction that the patients had with the overall health care service that they received.

Team Care in General Practice

Geoffrey Marsh and Peter Kaim-Caudle

Routledge
Taylor & Francis Group

First published in 1976 by Croom Helm Ltd.

This edition first published in 2026 by Routledge
4 Park Square, Milton Park, Abingdon, Oxon, OX14 4RN

and by Routledge
605 Third Avenue, New York, NY 10158

Routledge is an imprint of the Taylor & Francis Group, an informa business

ISBN: 978-1-041-33988-5 (hbk)
ISBN: 978-1-003-79052-5 (ebk)
ISBN: 978-1-041-33989-2 (pbk)

Book DOI 10.4324/9781003790525

TEAM CARE IN GENERAL PRACTICE

GEOFFREY MARSH
PETER KAIM-CAUDLE

With a Foreword by
PROFESSOR MARGOT JEFFERYS

CROOM HELM LONDON

First published 1976

Croom Helm Ltd, 2-10 St. John's Road, London, S.W.11.
ISBN 0 85664-153-7

Printed in Great Britain by Biddles of Guildford

CONTENTS

Forward 1

Part I The Workload Survey

1. General Practice Today 13
2. Variations in Workload 24
3. The Primary Health Care Team 34
4. A Profile of the Norton Practice 46
5. Disease Prevalence and Hospital Referrals 53
6. Facts and Figures 55
7. Low Workload – Satisfied Patients? 61

Appendix Mechanics of Data Collection 68

Tables 81

Part II The Patient Satisfaction Survey

8. The Survey 111
9. The Findings 119
10. Comments and Conclusions 129

Tables 141

Index 183

FOREWORD

By Margot Jefferys

When I was a school child in the inter-war years, my family lived in a small town within commuting distance of London. Our family doctor was one of two serving the district. His elegant house was in the High Street and he saw his private patients there. They walked through the front door to the comfortable waiting room. He had 'panel' patients – working class men for the most part – who were entitled to consult him by nature of their compulsory National Health Insurance payments. They entered by a side door where they waited in a long corridor for his services. Later, because the town grew and his practice thrived, he took on two assistants, a dispenser, and a shop a hundred yards or so down the street to which he transferred his panel but not his private practice. There was no nurse attached to his practice. The townsfolk criticised his wife for her unwillingness to play her socially expected role of receptionist and doctor's escort with female patients, and found it a blessing that his daughter, when she left school, was willing to do so. In the meantime, urgent messages were taken by one or other of the maids who graced his establishment. The well-to-do families had no hesitation in asking the doctor to call on them at home. It was they who decided whether a home visit was necessary and were billed for the privilege.

I suppose this type of practice was still to be found in some areas with a substantial number of middle class people when the National Health Service began in 1948, although the war may have blurred the crassest class distinctions. In more solidly working class areas the doctor was still likely to be a single-handed practitioner, but he was more likely for the sake of his wife and children to have moved his residence to a more salubrious part of the town while keeping his practice going in a shop close to his potential panel patients.

The patterns of primary medical care which I have recalled from my childhood were a reflection not only of the state of medical knowledge at the time, but also of the marked and largely unquestioned social divisions of a society which were mirrored in the medical care system. The divisions of that time have not altogether disappeared; but the impact of the second world war resulted at least in more egalitarian access to medical care. Changes since then in the economy, in technology, and in the life style expectations of individuals in all walks of life have combined to bring about a number of changes in the way in which medical services are organised.

Practices of the kind I recall from the inter-war years have not perhaps disappeared altogether. In 1973, the year in which the study reported in this book was undertaken, nearly a fifth of all principals in general practice under contract to the National Health Service in England and Wales were still in single-handed practice. Many of them survive, as did my family doctor 50 years ago, with the help of a succession of hard working assistants and a wife or daughter as receptionist. Some surgeries are probably no better equipped now than they were then and some of the loners are probably as remote from the local hub of the medical world – the hospital – and the prestigeful specialists as their forebears ever were.

But the general practitioner who works in isolation from his medical colleagues in the hospital or his peers in general practice in the locality is becoming a rarer bird even among single-handed practitioners. Younger recruits to this branch of medicine are now much more likely than those close to retirement age ever were to work in a colleaguely way with consultants and to seek out other general practitioners for the purpose of continuing their medical education in matters of both clinical and organisational interest.

Furthermore, group practice in or outside Health Centres, with attached Local (now Area) Health Authority workers as well as directly employed receptionists and secretarial staff, is now the most prevalent form of practice arrangement.

Most of these changes which have occurred in the structure of primary health care facilities and staffing in the last decade have not been described in much detail. There is little more than a few anecdotal accounts of the effects which such changes have had on the participants in the enterprise – that is, on doctors, other health and administative workers and – not least – on patients.

In particular, it is not at all clear what the results are of bringing doctors and nurses, including health visitors, together to provide potentially more comprehensive and coordinated community care for a patient population. The existence of a multi-professional team has at least the potential which isolated professionals have not of reallocating tasks in order to achieve the optimal distribution of work; but it is not clear how often this potential is utilised.

Of course the use of the word 'optimal' requires consideration. It is unlikely that the optimal distribution of tasks viewed from a particular perspective – for example that of the general practitioners – will be seen as optimal by all their patients, or all health visitors, or the government responsible to the tax payers for financing the service. In the harsh world of scarce resources and differential statuses accorded to those who possess different kinds of knowledge and skills, optimal solutions are likely to favour those who have the most power to command resources at the expense of those with least bargaining power. But no one is powerless and solutions can never be totally satisfactory, even for the most powerful, if only because those who feel dissatisfied with the role they have been allocated or with the rewards they obtain or with the services they receive have ways of making miserable the lives of those who dominate.

Fortunately too, power is not always used entirely egotistically. If it were, much less regard would be paid in the health service to the needs of the disadvantaged – the elderly infirm, the physically and mentally handicapped.

In this book Geoffrey Marsh and Peter Kaim-Caudle have tried to set out, honestly and clearly, what happened when the former made a deliberate attempt to reallocate tasks traditionally performed by the general practitioner to nurses and health visitors, while retaining the concept of the personal doctor. In part I the effect of bringing nurses into the consultative process – particularly in the home – on the workloads of all members of the practice and on referrals to hospital is discussed. Part II gives the results of a survey conducted independently by a team from the University of Durham of patients' reactions to the reallocation.

The story they have to tell is, by and large, a success story. The reallocation of tasks appears to have reduced the volume of work which the doctor undertook without increasing the work referred to specialists. Other members of the health care team appear to have been pleased to accept more clinical responsibility; and patients, although not uncritical of some aspects of practice organisation, did not complain about the care they received from nurses. The third party too, the state, should have reason to be pleased, for one implication of the study was the finding (to be confirmed more generally) that manpower demands for community health care can be curtailed if small multi-professional teams are encouraged to take on work hitherto performed purely by medically qualified personnel.

Nevertheless, the authors are rightly cautious. They did not attempt to measure the vexatious issue of the quality of the care delivered. However unlikely, it is conceivable, that if we were able to devise satisfactory ways of measuring the effects of care on the health experience of the population, delegation of some physicians' tasks to nurses could be shown to be deleterious. Similarly, we cannot say whether patient satisfaction would be as great given another practitioner. Innovations have a way of being successful because innovators are thoughtful people with charisma and enthusiasm. It will be for the future historians of medical care to assess the significance of the pioneering work which is so faithfully recorded here.

ACKNOWLEDGEMENTS

We acknowledge with gratitude the following people who have helped us in the writing of this book:

Richard Burnett for compiling statistics in Part II.

Janice Casey for reading and amending the text.

Audrey Denton for being a most perseverant research secretary.

Margaret Hammond, Librarian, Royal College of General Practitioners, for help with the references.

Margot Jefferys for help with the patient satisfaction questionnaire and for contributing the foreword.

Michael Jenkins and Mark Johnson for computing in Part II.

Beverley Kimble, USA, 'Rotary' scholar at Durham University, 1972-3, for leading the survey team.

Kathleen McFarlane for typing and assembling the manuscript.

Angus McNay for the statistics in Part I.

THE NEWCASTLE-UPON-TYNE REGIONAL HOSPITAL BOARD for two research grants.

THE PARTNERS and all the members of the Primary Health Care Team in the Norton practice for painstaking recording throughout the survey year.

And not least our wives whose constant support and encouragement is our greatest strength.

P. R. KAIM-CAUDLE
G. N. MARSH

PART I THE WORKLOAD SURVEY

1 GENERAL PRACTICE TODAY

The Trend Towards Group Practice

A recently qualified doctor entering general practice today will find a very different environment from that which his counterpart experienced only ten years ago. Increasingly, he is likely to join a Primary Health Care Team in a purpose-built medical centre. Over the last decade, there has been a pronounced movement towards large group practices with supporting professional and lay staff and the cramped single-handed practice attached to the doctor's home with little or no secretarial or nursing help is becoming extinct. The rate of change has been rapid since 1966, the year in which the numerous recommendations of the BMA's family doctor charter were accepted by the British Government. [1] Some of these changes have greatly affected the doctor's workload and have important implications for the future. The increase in the number and variety of staff employed by practices, the evolution of the Primary Health Care Team, and the attachment of local authority staff (area health authority staff after April 1974) to practices have had noteworthy effects which will be discussed in detail.

Less than a fifth of general practitioners now work in single-handed practices and a new doctor will normally expect to join a group of three or more. [2] The concept of group practice was put forward as long ago as 1920 in the Dawson Report, which suggested that doctors should work in teams from health centres. [3] During the last twenty years, opinion in favour of groups has gathered momentum, but there is still disagreement about the optimum size of a group. Taylor, in 1954, advocated the system of group practice in his book, *Good General Practice* [4] and this view was supported nine years later by the Gillie Report. [5] The Royal Commission on Medical Education (1968) suggested that groups of at least a dozen doctors would have economic and professional advantages and would benefit patients. [6] The Sub-Committee of the Standing Medical Advisory Committee on the Organisation of Group Practice concluded in 1971 that the optimum size for groups would prove to be five or six doctors. [7]

The British Medical Association's Planning Unit Report of 1970 put the case for larger groups succinctly when stating, 'Our subjective judgement accords with Cartwright's [8] findings that, on the whole, doctors in larger units derive greater satisfaction from their work than those working in single-handed or in two-man partnerships. [9] We believe that this is due to the opportunity afforded to use more of their professional skills by delegation of work to medically related workers and to generally improved working conditions.'

It is now generally accepted that the newly qualified doctor needs to undergo a period of training in general practice before he can become a principal, and the presence of these trainees itself increases the size of the group. In 1967 the number of trainee practitioners in England and Wales had fallen to 120 but by October 1972 it had risen to 315. [10] By October 1974 there were not less than 460 trainee places available in recognised three-year package schemes. [11] If training becomes compulsory about 1,000 places will be required. [6]

The rise in the number of doctors working in group practices has kept pace with opinion in favour of these groups. The number of large partnerships has steadily increased. In 1958, as many as 33 per cent of all general practitioners were single-handed. By 1972 this proportion had fallen to 19 per cent. Conversely, in 1958 only 5 per cent of practices had five or six doctors but by 1972 this had risen to 15 per cent.[2]

New Medical Centres

The trend towards larger practices has been one of the factors leading to the realisation that larger and different types of medical centres are desirable. The family doctor charter encouraged two types – the local authority health centre and the group practice centre. [1]

After 1966, the Ministry of Health approved plans for local authority health centres only if they provided facilities for general practitioners. The number of these centres has greatly increased since 1969 when fifty were opened. Three years later 10 per cent of all general practitioners worked from 365 health centres in England [12] and the Chief Medical Officer of the Department of Health and Social Security estimated that by the end of 1974 500 health centres would be operational with one in seven general practitioners working from them. [13]

The responsibility for the design, building and maintenance of these premises rested with the local health authorities (regional health authorities after April 1974). They were guided by the Department of Health and Social Security publication (1970) – '*Health Centres – a Design Guide*'. [14] The health centre programme did not require any capital contribution from general practitioners. Furthermore, they were reimbursed the rents which they paid for the use of facilities within the centre by the executive councils (family practitioner committees of the area health authorities after April 1974).

The proportion of doctors working from group practice centres which they have provided for themselves is much greater than that working from health centres. Group practice centres are either expansions of existing surgeries or new purpose-built premises to accommodate the doctors and their teams. Although the doctors themselves are responsible for the planning, building and maintenance of these premises, they liaise with the local authorities in the provision of facilities for attached staff. The Design Guide to Group Practice Centres published by the Ministry of Health in 1966, assists general practitioners in the building, improving and expanding of premises. [15]

The capital cost of these centres is the responsibility of the doctors but they are helped by the General Practice Finance Corporation which was established in 1967 to make long-term loans for the building of such centres. [16] The corporation charges commercial rates of interest – 16 per cent in 1974. [17] It made 1,840 loans to 3,837 doctors between 1967 and March 1973 and the total sum lent was £12,266,000. [18] The doctors are paid rent for the premises they provide which is assessed by the district valuer and paid by the executive council (family practitioner committee after April 1974). On new purpose-built premises the rent is guaranteed at a level which will equal the interest rates charged by the General Practice Finance Corporation. [19]

Furthermore, groups who are improving their existing premises are eligible for a 30 per cent non-repayable grant. [20] Almost 2,000 grants totalling approximately £850,000 have been paid in England and Wales between 1966 and 1973. [12] Irrespective of the accommodation which they occupy, general practitioners working in groups receive as part of their annual remuneration a group practice allowance of £270 (in 1974). [21] The purpose of this allowance is to encourage the formation of group practices.

Irvine and Jefferys' (1971) postal survey showed that most *young* doctors were working in groups and that a large proportion were working from local authority health centres. [22] With a few notable exceptions, these centres provided more space, equipment and staff than other premises. Groups in privately owned centres tended to make more effective use of their premises and staff. They spent a larger proportion of the money available to them on their practices and used appointment systems more often. Nearly 33 per cent of these doctors still had their premises attached to their own or their partner's houses. Many of these premises were lacking in space, a finding which underlined the need for a large rebuilding programme.

Irvine's survey (1972) of 190 teaching practices (training newly qualified doctors) found that 75 per cent used premises which were owned by a group of partnership and that only 12 per cent worked from local authority health centres; the other 13 per cent occupied premises which were owned by private landlords. [23] Amongst these teaching doctors, 17 per cent worked in premises attached to their own or their partners' houses.

The Primary Health Care Team

The trend towards larger group practices and the resultant improvement in accommodation has been an important factor in the increase of staff working with the doctors and sharing their premises and work load.

There are marked variations in the structure of these teams. Some are in the early, formative stages while others are more fully developed. It is the evolution of this team of workers which has most revolutionised general practice today. It is to have repercussions both on the kind of care which patients are coming to expect and on the workload of the doctor.

A highly developed team now consists of a group of general practitioners and trainee doctors working together with nurses, health visitors, midwives, receptionists, secretaries and filing clerks. It will usually have some form of liaison with social workers from the Department of Social Services in the area. Some teams also liaise with such agencies as the Family Planning Association, the Samaritans, the Marriage Guidance Council and the local clergy, but this is not common. Student nurses, trainee health visitors and pupil midwives all form part of the fully functioning team. All midwives and health visitors as well as most of the nurses are in the employment of the area health authority, which attaches them to doctors' practices. The Board of Science and Education of the British Medical Association have recently produced a monograph on such Primary Health Care Teams. [24]

Secretarial Staff

The doctors employ their own secretarial staff, a term which embraces all clerical, secretarial and administrative workers in practices. In 1971 a sub-committee of the Standing Medical Advisory Committee on the organisation of group practice [6] advocated that as much clerical work and routine administration as possible should be delegated to secretarial staff so that general practitioners could make full use of their professional training. It went further in suggesting that secretarial assistance should also be provided for nurses, health visitors and social workers so that they also could use their special skills to the full. The need for four kinds of worker was recognised – receptionists, record clerks, medical typists and practice managers. It is now easier for doctors to implement these recommendations since, following the family doctor charter, [1] the family practitioner committee reimburses 70 per cent of the wages of secretarial staff. The Department of Health and Social Security has, however, ruled that this reimbursement should only apply to the equivalent of two full-time employees per doctor, and that their work must not include research or educational activities. [21]

Irvine and Jefferys (1971) [22] reported that as many as 97 per cent of the practices in their sample employed some secretarial staff – 38 per cent two, and 60 per cent more than four staff. This was a considerable improvement compared with a similar survey eight years earlier when only 66 per cent of practices had any secretarial assistance. [25] Drury and Kuenssberg nevertheless concluded, as recently as 1970, that many doctors did not delegate clerical and routine duties appropriately to secretarial staff. [26]

In 1969 the North-West Merseyside faculty of the Royal College of General Practitioners presented the results of a postal questionnaire which showed that there was no relationship between the number of hours of clerical work a practice used each week and the total number of patients registered with the practice, the number of patients on individual doctors' lists, or the number of doctors in the group. [27] They did find, however, that those practices which used more clerical assistance were more likely to have an appointment system. Irvine (1972) found that teaching practices had more secretarial assistance than the practices in the Merseyside survey.[23] A quarter of the teaching doctors in his sample had over sixteen hours of secretarial help per 1,000 patients per week.

It is important that secretarial staff should receive adequate training if they are to play their full part in the running of the practice. This is especially true if these staff are to carry some of the workload which has previously been undertaken by the doctor. This need is now acknowledged and is being met. Courses for receptionists and secretaries were recommended by the sub-committee of the Standing Medical Advisory Committee [6] in 1971 and the need for training and education of such staff re-emphasised in 1974 by the Department of Health and Social Security joint working party report on general medical services. [28] A training syllabus has been devised by the Association of Medical Secretaries and an increasing number of technical colleges are offering courses. [29] *The Medical Secretaries' Handbook* gives helpful guidance to secretarial and receptionist staff. [30]

Nurses

Many doctors also employ their own nurses. Their salaries like those of the secretarial staff, can be reimbursed up to 70 per cent by the family practitioner committee. The employment of nurses by general practitioners has been studied fairly comprehensively [31, 32, 33, 34, 35, 36] and has pioneered the development of local authority attachment schemes. In the past local authority nurses provided care for patients within a defined geographical area and were known as district nurses. This ended with the attachment of these nurses to particular practices.

The growth of these attachment schemes has been dramatic. From 1968 to 1969 the number of local authority nurses working in general practice attachment schemes more than doubled, the proportion rising from 11 to 24 per cent. [37] By 1973 the proportion had increased sevenfold and 77 per cent of all nurses were attached. However, even then almost a quarter of all local authority nurses were still unattached. These statistics are consistent with Irvine's findings that a fifth of his sample of teaching doctors had no nursing staff working with them.[23]

The report of the Joint Working Party on Attachment of Nursing Services to General Practice (1970) considered that ideally all nurses should be employed by the local authority and thought it undesirable for nurses working in the same practice to have different employers.[38] However, it was conceded that the shortage of local authority nurses did not make this practicable. General practitioners still have to employ their own nurses since many of them do not benefit from attachment schemes. Even practices which do have such schemes may also need their own nursing staff if they are to receive adequate assistance, and especially if they wish to have a nurse available at the surgery throughout the day.

Various and conflicting estimates have been made of the number of nurses required by each doctor's practice. Such estimates are often expressed as the number of hours of nurse work per 1,000 patients per week. The Gillie Report (1963) [5] postulated one full-time nurse for a four-doctor group practice or about four hours per 1,000 patients per week. A similar conclusion was reached by the Royal College of General Practitioners' study of four north-eastern practices in 1968. [39] The Joint Working Party on Attachment of Nursing Services to General Practice (1970) made no estimate of the number of hours' work which it considered desirable. [38] The sub-committee of the Standing Medical Advisory Committee (1971) was more specific and recommended eight hours of state registered nurse's time per 1,000 patients per week. [6] This happened to correspond with the number of nurses available at the time they reported.

The many studies of nurse attachment schemes convey a fairly clear picture of the amount of work nurses do in various practices but they are deficient in discussing what is theoretically desirable. Nor do they always report the exact tasks which were assigned to nurses. Some of the differences in the number of hours worked in the reporting practices may well reflect the variety of tasks performed.

Warin's report (1968) is particularly interesting as it is the first account of a complete attachment scheme. [40] His scheme in Oxford was completed before schemes had even started in many other areas. In 1963 he attached one district nurse to a three-doctor group and two years later all the nurses in Oxford were attached to general practices. One nurse was provided for every 5,200 patients which represented seven and a half hours' nurse time per 1,000 patients per week. Warin recognises the need for larger practices to have a nurse working at the practice centre so that attached nurses can concentrate on home visiting.

Weston Smith and Donovan (1970), who initiated the system of nurses making the first contact with sick patients at home, surprisingly employed their own nurses for only three hours per 1,000 patients per week. [41] In contrast, Hasler *et al*(1966) had both a district nurse and a nurse's auxiliary for their 6,800 patients as well as employing two part-time nursing sisters to provide full-time treatment roomcover. [42] This amounted to as much as twelve hours' work per 1,000 patients per week.

The North-West Merseyside study (1969) found that practices employing their own nurses in addition to attached nurses had the highest number of nurse-working hours per 1,000 patients.[27] A third of the practices had attached staff only and achieved an average of four and a half hours per 1,000 patients per week, whereas the 11 per cent of practices employing both private and local authority nurses achieved an average of nearly seven hours per 1,000 patients per week. Dixon's study in a small Bristol health centre (1969) led him to suggest that six hours of nursing time per 1,000 patients per week were required solely for work in the treatment room.[43]

Howard (1970), herself a nurse, described the attachment scheme in which she was working in Birmingham. She worked full-time for a population of 8,300, or nearly five hours per 1,000 patients per week.[44] She was supported by a full-time state enrolled nurse. Law (1970) studied ten urban group practices in the South of England each serving 12,000 patients.[45] Every practice contained a doctor who had either published work on general practice or was on a committee concerned with the improvement of general practice. Although the average number of hours was five per 1,000 patients per week, the range was from none at all to over thirteen. Irvine's study found that 31 per cent of teaching practices had between one and five hours of nurses' time, 22 per cent had between six and ten hours, 12 per cent had between eleven and fifteen hours, and 6 per cent had between sixteen and twenty hours per 1,000 patients per week.[23]

Health Visitors

Whereas the attachment of local authority nurses to practices was a fairly natural development from the employment of nurses by the doctors themselves, there was no precedent for the employment of health visitors. Indeed the true role of the health visitor was not appreciated by many general practitioners, who had a very vague idea of her knowledge and skills. There was normally little or no personal contact between these two professions, communication being limited to an occasional telephone call or, more frequently, to notes or messages brought to the doctor by patients from local authority child welfare clinics. These messages frequently suggested treatment with which the general practitioner disagreed. This may have been due to the fact that the health visitors worked at their clinics with assistant medical officers of health whose knowledge, attitudes and traditions were often very different from those of the general practitioner.

In the years preceding the introduction of attachment schemes some nurses employed by general practitioners did work, such as immunisation schemes and well-baby clinics, which is traditionally assigned to health visitors.[31] This was to lead to some confusion between the roles of the nurse and the health visitor in the primary health care team.

Published reports on the employment of nurses in general practices played an important part in guiding local authorities in the early days of nurse attachment schemes. Donaldson, for example, deliberately began his attachment scheme in Teesside by attaching nurses to practices because nurses and doctors were already cooperative partners with a mature understanding of each other's role. [46] Three doctors in his area had published work on the nurses employed by their practices. [31, 36, 39] In contrast, local authorities had no guidance from reports on the employment of health visitors.

There was another difficulty. The role of the health visitor in education and counselling depended to an appreciable extent on her relationship with the whole family. The fact that different members of the same same family are often registered with different practices could lead to confusion when the health visitor is attached to only one practice. [47] Despite these problems, once the attachment of health visitors to practices had commenced it grew as quickly as the attachment of nurses. [48, 49, 50, 51, 52, 53] By 1970 half the health visitors in England and Wales were attached and by 1973 the proportion had risen to 78 per cent, about the same as that of district nurses. [12]

Some areas are extremely short of health visitors and experience great difficulties in recruitment while others are more fortunate. This makes the range in the number of hours worked by health visitors per 1,000 patients per week as great as that worked by nurses. Various studies present a picture of the situation in different parts of the country. In the early days of attachment, Fry *et al* (1965) described the work of a health visitor serving the 7,500 patients in their practice. [48] A survey in three urban areas of Hertfordshire (1968) following the attachment of health visitors to practices showed that the health visitors' patient population varied from 1,000 to 5,000. [54] Warin in Oxford attached one health visitor for every 5,700 patients, but made the important point that the number of patients alone is not a reliable guide to the amount of work generated. [40] For example, one practice of 5,000 patients on a new housing estate contained many small children and therefore required two health visitors, while a practice of 9,000 patients near the university needed only one. He also noted that areas with a large proportion of immigrants or old people had a greater need for health visitors.

The North-West Merseyside study revealed a very different situation from that in Oxford.[27] Only one third of the practices had any work at all done by a health visitor, 17 per cent used a health visitor for three or more hours per 1,000 patients per week, 7 per cent for two to three hours and 17 per cent for less than two hours. In Law's study one health visitor served an average of 8,000 patients but there were considerable variations from one for 4,000 to one for 16,000 patients. [45]

Irvine found that 71 per cent of his sample of doctors in teaching practices had health visitors attached. [23] In 6 per cent of the practices the health visitor worked six hours per 1,000 patients per week, in

31 per cent one to five hours, and in 24 per cent over six hours.

These studies led the Chief Medical Officer of Health of the Department of Health and Social Security to suggest in his annual report for 1971 that a ratio of one health visitor to every 4,000 patients was desirable. [55] In the same year the Standing Medical Advisory Committee considered one health visitor for every two principals in a group as a realistic assessment, having regard to the number of health visitors available. Nevertheless the great majority of practices have inadequate numbers of health visitors. Moreover the role and range of her responsibilities within the Primary Health Care Team is still ill defined.

Midwives

At the end of 1970, 15 per cent of local authority midwives were attached to practices. [37] However, there are very few studies of such attachements [56,57] possibly because doctors and midwives always have and still do work together whether or not formal attachment has taken place. Warin attached midwives in pairs to practices, providing on average one midwife for every six to eight doctors, depending on the amount of obstetric work available. [40] Most areas of England and Wales with a significant amount of obstetric work put their midwives on a comprehensive rota system, as labours and deliveries extend across on- and off-duty periods. This arrangement is necessary whether midwives are attached or not. For this reason most midwives have a fairly equal delivery workload, but those attached will undertake a variable amount of ante-natal care, depending on the amount of obstetric work in the practice.

Little guidance regarding the attachment of midwives has been provided by any official body. The report of the joint working party makes almost no reference to this subject beyond suggesting that attachment of midwives should take place. [38] The Standing Medical Advisory Committee [6] supports the recommendation of the Peel report that nearly all women should have their babies in hospital. [58] It envisaged, however, that the hospital midwife should also be a member of the Primary Health Care Team. With over 90 per cent of births now taking place in hospital and the average in-patient stay about six days a closer integration of hospital and domiciliary services has important implications for the role of the midwife.

The attachment of midwives to general practice is now widely favoured and is proceeding steadily, but the attachment of local authority nurses and health visitors is still more frequent and has had a more dramatic impact on the workload of the general practitioner.

Notes

1. British Medical Association (1965) *A Charter for the Family Doctor Service.*
2. Department of Health and Social Security *Digest of Health Statistics – England and Wales 1973.* HMSO, London.

3. Dawson Report (1920) *Interim Report of the Consultative Council on Future Provision of Medical and Allied Services*.HMSO, London.
4. Taylor, S. (1954) *Good General Practice*. Oxford University Press, London.
5. *The Field of Work of the Family Doctor* (Gillie Report) (1963). HMSO, London.
6. *Report of the Royal Commission on Medical Education,* (1968). HMSO, London.
7. Department of Health and Social Security Welsh Office (1971) *Organisation of Group Practice,* A report of the Sub-Committee of the Standing Medical Advisory Committee. HMSO, London.
8. Cartwright, A. (1967) *Patients and their Doctors.* Routledge and Kegan Paul, London.
9. British Medical Association (1970) Planning Unit Report No. 4, Primary Medical Care.
10. Wintersgill, W. (1973) Recruitment of unrestricted principals in general practice. *Health Trends,* 5, 2, 26-7.
11. Horder, J.P. The trainee year. Letter in *Brit. Med. J.,*1975, 2, 142.
12. Department of Health and Social Security (1973) Annual Report of the Chief Medical Officer. *On the State of the Public Health.* HMSO, London.
13. Chief Medical Officer, Notes from *Health Trends,* 72, 4, 1, 1.
14. Department of Health and Social Security (1970) *Health Centres – a Design Guide.* HMSO, London.
15. College of General Practitioners, (1966) *A Design Guide for Medical Group Practice Centres.*
16. *Report of General Practice Finance Corporation* (1967). HMSO, London.
17. General Practice Finance Corporation Letter to family practitioner committees and area health authority, 28 August 1974.
18. *Report of General Practice Finance Corporation* (1974). HMSO, London.
19. Executive Council Notice 1019 *Direct Payment Scheme for Rent and Rates.*
20. Executive Council Notice 621. *Improvement Grants.*
21. Department of Health and Social Security Welsh Office. *Statement of Fees and Allowances payable to General Medical Practitioners in England and Wales.*
22. Irvine, D. and Jefferys, M. (1971) British Medical Association Planning Unit Survey of General Practice, 1969. *Brit. Med. J.,* 1971, 4, 535-43.
23. Irvine, D. (1972) Reports from general practice. No.15, *Teaching Practices, Royal College of General Practitioners* 1972.
24. British Medical Association, Board of Science and Education (1974) *Report of the Panel on Primary Health Care Teams.*
25. Cartwright, A. and Marshall, R. (1965) General Practice in 1963. *Medical Care,* 3, 69.
26. Drury, M. and Kuenssberg, E.V. (1970) General practice observed. *Brit. Med. J.,* 1970, 4, 42-4.
27. Royal College of General Practitioners (1970) Symposium on General Practice, *North-West Merseyside Survey.*
28. Department of Health and Social Security (1974) *Report of the Joint Working Party: General Medical Services*.HMSO, London.
29. Association of Medical Secretaries (1971) London: *Examination Syllabus for Diploma and Certificate for Medical Secretaries.*
30. Drury, M. (1965) *The Medical Secretaries' Handbook.* Bailliere, Tindall & Cassell, London.
31. Marsh, G.N. (1967) Group practice nurse: an analysis and comment on six months' work. *Brit. Med. J.,* 1967, i, 489-91.

32. Baldwin, J.T. (1967) The use of the nurse in general practice. *Jnl. Coll. Gen. Pract.*, 1967, 13, 364-7.
33. Hodgkin, G.K.H. (1967) Saving doctor's time with a practice nurse. Conference: *The Team. Family Health Care*, 1967.
34. Murray, J. (1967) Fifteen years in general practice. *Jnl. R.C.G.P.*, 1967, 13, 367-72.
35. Weston Smith, J. and Mottramm, E.M. (1967) Extended use of nursing services in general practice. *Brit. Med. J.*, 1967, 4, 672-4.
36. Marsh, G.N. (1969) Visiting nurse – analysis of one year's work. *Brit. Med. J.*, 1969, 4, 42-4.
37. Anderson, J.A.D. *et al* (1970) Attachment of community nurses to general practices. A follow-up study. *Brit. Med. J.*, 1970, 4, 103-5.
38. Department of Health and Social Security (1970) *Report of Joint Working Party on Group Attachment. Attachment of Nursing Services in General Practice.* HMSO, London.
39. Royal College of General Practitioners (1968) *The Practice Nurse.* Reports from General Practice, No. 10, 1968.
40. Warin, J.F. (1968) General practitioners and nursing staff: a complete attachment scheme in retrospect and prospect. *Brit. Med. J.*, 1968, 2, 41-5.
41. Weston Smith, J. and Donovan, J.B. (1970) The practice nurse – a new look. *Brit. Med. J.*, 1970, 4, 637-77.
42. Hasler, J.C. *et al* (1972) Training for the treatment room sister in general practice. *Brit. Med. J.*, 1972, 1, 232-4.
43. Dixon, P.M. (1969) Work of a nurse in a health centre treatment room. *Brit. Med. J.*, 1969, 4, 292-4.
44. Howard, A.L. (1970) Twelve months' attachment: from the local authority. *Nursing Times*, 1970, 66, 1390-1.
45. Law, R. (1970) Communication and cooperation within the primary health team. *Jnl. R.C.G.P.*, 1970, 20, 6-12.
46. Donaldson, R.J. (1971) Personal communication.
47. Watson, C. and Clark, M. (1972) Attachment schemes and development of the Health Team. *Update*, 1972, 4, 489-94.
48. Fry, J. *et al* (1965) The evolution of a health team: a successful general practitioner-health visitor attachment. *Brit. Med. J.*, 1965, 1, 181-3.
49. Williamson, J. *et al* (1966) The use of health visitors in preventative geriatrics. *Geront. Clin.*, 1966, 8, 362-9.
50. Lewis, T.D. (1968) Health visitor and the family doctor. *Jnl. R.C.G.P.*, 1968, 15, 241-3.
51. Parish, P.A. (1968) Health visitor attachment in general practice. *Nursing Times*, 1968, 64, 256-9.
52. Hattersley, F.G. (1968) Health visitor attachments. *Practitioner*, 1968, 200, 422-6.
53. Ness, M.T. and Reekie, M.M. (1970) Old people in group practice. *Nursing Times*, 1970, 66, 1232-3.
54. Allen, W.H. and King, V.M. (1968) A study of health visitor attachments to general practitioners in Hertfordshire. *Medical Officer*, 1968, 119, 177-80.
55. Department of Health and Social Security (1971) Annual Report of the Chief Medical Officer. *On the state of the Public Health.* HMSO, London.
56. Donaldson, R.J. (1970) *Teach-in on team work.* Teesside Health Department, 1970.
57. Burn, J.L. (1971) New horizons in team work. *Practitioner*, 1971, 206, 801-6.
58. *Domiciliary Midwifery and Maternity Bed Needs* (Peel Report) (1970). HMSO, London.

2. VARIATIONS IN WORKLOAD

Consultation Rates

Doctors' workloads vary very considerably. Any doctor will find himself with more work on a Monday morning in February than on a fine Friday afternoon in September. Variations in workload between different doctors depend on factors as unrelated as the proportion of elderly patients on their lists and the attitude of individual doctors to home visiting. To put the detailed study of the doctors' workload in a particular practice into perspective, it is necessary to survey several studies of practices which have been undertaken in this country during the last twenty years.

The assessment of the doctor's workload is normally based on the average number of consultations which he has with each registered patient during the year. The term 'consultation' has been defined as 'an occasion on which a patient receives professional advice or help or treatment from his doctor' and this is the sense in which it will be used here.[1] This definition presupposes face-to-face contact between patient and doctor and thus excludes telephone conversations, repeat prescriptions for continuing illnesses, or prescriptions for new illnesses whose symptoms or signs are reported to the doctor by a third party.

The average number of consultations per patient per year in Great Britain is not known for certain. Logan and Cushion (1958) in their review of 106 practices found an average rate of nearly four consultations per year.[2] Cartwright (1967) however, pointed out that these practices were not necessarily typical as they had not been randomly selected and that particular consultation rate was lower than normal.[3] In her own study 1,400 patients were interviewed and from this she derived an average rate of four and a half per patient per year. She considered that this may have been an underestimate as it relied on patients' recollections which may have been faulty. She concluded that the average consultation rate for England and Wales was probably five. The regional medical officers undertook a survey of 3,000 doctors during 1964-5 and recorded an average consultation rate of five and a half consultations.[4] The General Household Survey for 1973 put the average rate much lower at 3.8.[5]

A characteristic of workload studies is the very wide variation in the consultation rate between different practices. Logan and Cushion reported a variation of between three and nine consultations per patient per year.[2] The Royal College of General Practitioners reported rates varying from three to seven, some general practitioners having twice as many consultations per patient as others.[6] Williams (1970) reported that in a large South Wales survey the average number of consultations per patient per year varied from three to ten,[7] and Wright (1968) found variations of between two and eight in a similar survey in south-west England.[8]

Fry's study (1970) of twelve general practices also revealed a wide variation despite the fact that these practices were workload-orientated and therefore had low average consultation rates.[6] Average surgery attendances varied from two to four and a half per patient per year, while average home visits varied from a half to nearly two.

The ratio of surgery attendances to home visits has become an important criterion in assessing the doctor's workload. Doctors make fewer home visits than they did in the past and Fry could find no evidence that this had led to an increase in the number of attendances at the surgery;[6] it is consequently reasonable to assume that the doctor's workload has decreased. The surgery attendance/home visit ratio (A/V ratio) has been recorded in many studies and will be noted in discussing the factors which have been found to affect the general practitioner's workload.

Geographical Area

One such factor is the area in which the practice is located. Heavy industry and atmospheric pollution are associated with high morbidity and in such areas a high consultation rate is to be expected. Posner (1965) stresses this point and reports a rate of five consultations from Sunderland in the industrial north-east.[9] Williams, in his study of South Wales, found that mining areas had the highest consultation rate – six and a half per patient per year.[7] The average consultation rate over the area as a whole was five and a half which contrasts with the lower rate of four in south-west England.[8] Williams concluded that this difference was largely due to the prevalence of serious cardio-respiratory disease in the area of South Wales which he studied.

All general practitioners working in mining areas report high consultation rates.[7, 10, 11, 12] Logan (1958) found the consultation rate for miners to be two to three times that of other occupational groups.[2] This is partly due to the arduous nature of the miner's work which prevents him working when he suffers from a comparatively minor illness and partly due to the exceptionally high accident rate in the mining industry.[13] The analysis of sickness certificates by the Ministry of Pensions and National Insurance confirms the high incidence of sickness amongst miners.

In high-density town areas there are generally fewer home visits than in rural areas. Williams found that while the consultation rate in mining areas was very high, there were proportionally fewer home visits in these areas than in the rural areas of his study.[7] He reported a ratio of surgery attendances to home visits of four to one for mining areas and of two to one in country towns and rural areas. Wright, in the south-west, reported a ratio of two attendances to one home visit in country practices but three to one in town practices.[8] The greater frequency of home visits in country areas was also noted in Marsh *et al's* study of the north-east of England.[14]

The lower population density and the longer time required for home visiting in rural areas are generally accepted as the reasons why country doctors have fewer patients on their lists than town doctors. Studies confirm that a patient who lives some distance from the surgery not only involves the doctor in extra travelling time when he receives a home visit but also that he is more likely to ask for one. Hopkins *et al* (1968) in a study of their practice on the outskirts of Liverpool found that those patients who lived between three-quarters of a mile and two miles from the practice received a disproportionately larger number of home visits than those who lived nearer to the practice centre.[15] Longmore (1967) found that the 60 per cent of the patients of his Scottish practice who lived over three miles from the surgery had as many home visits as surgery attendances.[16]

In marked contrast to less densely populated areas Morrell's studies (1970) in central London show that distance from the surgery does not necessarily lead to a high proportion of home visits.[17] He found that the proportion of home visits to surgery attendances declined the further away the patient lived. He attributed this to the difficulty of visiting in an area of high traffic congestion. His practice had the exceptionally high ratio of surgery attendances to home visits of ten to one.

Many doctors limit the distance they are prepared to travel to see patients and occasional attempts have been made to reduce mileage in established but over-stretched practices. Thus Marsh (1968) reported that his group practice transferred 800 patients from its list because the distance they lived from the surgery made it difficult for them to attend, as well as causing the doctor a disproportionate amount of travelling time.[18] In Aberdeen several practices have used maps of patient distribution in order to work out a rational policy for practice catchment areas.[19]

It has been suggested that good transport facilities – private, public or special – are essential if the number of home visits is to be reduced. Marsh *et al* (1972) concluded that the provision of minibus transport for patients would reduce the need for home visits very appreciably, especially those to the chronically sick in rural areas.[14] Smith and Seddon (1968), who had a high proportion of elderly people in their practice, reduced their home visits by using a car to bring patients to the surgery.[20] Binnie (1970) found that car ownership was an important factor in determining whether patients would come to the surgery.[21] Lance's monograph (1971) on transport services confirmed that a larger proportion of consultations took place at the surgery in all practices where special transport was provided.[22] However, she leaves the reader with the impression that on account of the high cost she did not foresee such services being extended.

List Size

List size is another factor which might be expected to have an effect on the doctor's workload. The average number of patients on a doctor's list in England and Wales was 2,421 in 1972.[23] This figure has varied slightly over the years. Between 1958 and 1967 the average number rose from 2,269 to 2,479 as the recruitment to general practice failed to keep pace with the rapid increase in population which was largely caused by an increase in the number of births. Thereafter, recruitment improved mainly due to more doctors from overseas and more women entering general practice.[24]

Despite the efforts of the medical practices committee to bring about a more even distribution of doctors, there are still great variations in the list sizes of doctors in different parts of the country. They differ between areas by almost 1,000 patients. As has already been noted, country doctors tend to have smaller lists than doctors in more populated areas. This is partly because of operational reasons and low density of population, but may not be quite unconnected with the fact that some doctors prefer to live in rural surroundings.

It has been shown that variations in list size do have an effect on the doctor's aggregate workload. Wright found that in south-west England list sizes were inversely correlated to consultation rates.[8] Doctors with lists of less than 2,000 had an average annual consultation rate of nearly five, those with lists of 2,000 to 3,000 had a rate of four and those with over 3,000 patients had an average of three and a half consultations. The high consultation rate for doctors with small lists could not be accounted for by a higher proportion of follow-up consultations. Wright concluded that the discrepancy was due to a subtle difference in the doctor-patient relationship upon whose nature he could only speculate. Richardson (1973) in Aberdeen also found that the smaller the list size the higher the consultation rate.[25] Unlike Wright, however, he found that the smaller the list the greater was the proportion of consultations initiated by the doctor rather than the patient.

Size of partnership has no consistent effect on workload. Williams found that in South Wales groups of three or more doctors averaged over five consultations while two-men practices averaged nearly seven.[7] It may be that this difference is due to other factors quite unconnected with the size of group. Wright in the south-west did not find any correlation between consultation rate and number of doctors in a group.[8]

Appointment Systems

Appointment systems appear to have a more positive effect on workload. In both the South Wales and the south-west England studies, practices which had an appointment system showed, on average, about one consultation per patient per year less than those without appointment systems.[7,8] There was however a difference in the findings relating to the proportion of home visits: an appointment system made virtually no difference in the south-west of England but it was associated with a slightly higher ratio of attendances to home visits in South Wales.

The Doctor's Attitude

The patient has a more direct relationship with the doctor himself than with his practice. It is therefore relevant to enquire whether the attitude of the doctor towards his patients and their consultations affects his workload. Cartwright found that 70 per cent of the doctors she interviewed agreed that 'a good general practitioner can train his patients not to make unreasonable and unnecessary demands on his time'.[3] This is the subjective view of these doctors and impossible to verify, though this does not mean that it is untrue. The doctor's personality, ideology, motivation, and general interest in his job and his patients are also relevant and important but cannot be quantified. A doctor's policy of encouraging his patients to come back for further consultation will affect his workload. In Aberdeen this was the reason why doctors with smaller lists had higher consultation rates.[25] Richardson *et al* (1973) reported wide differences in the proportion of return consultation rates, with an average of 56 per cent. They concluded that the attitude of the individual doctor was the main cause for this.

Williams found that half the total consultations in his South Wales study were follow-ups.[7] He noted that the higher the rate of consultations initiated by patients, the lower the rate of consultations initiated by doctors. There were more follow-up consultations in rural areas. In south-west England there was a higher average follow-up rate of 58 per cent, again with a higher-than-average rate in rural areas.[8] Morrell in central London initiated only 47 per cent of his consultations.[17]

Marsh (1968) ascribed the decrease in the number of home visits in his practice from 1960 to 1967 largely to the attitude of the doctor.[18] He attributed the decline partly to his own increased personal experience coupled with a greater knowledge of his patients and their illnesses. His own attitude to home-visiting had changed – he considered it unnecessarily time-and energy-consuming for the results achieved, and attempted to educate his patients to use the surgery when ill rather than to stay in bed, to understand the course of their illnesses, and to time their visits to the surgery accordingly.

Age of Doctor and Patients

The age of the doctor affects workload. Both Wright and Williams found that the consultation rate declined as doctors became older.[7,8] The difference between doctors of under forty and those over fifty were consistent but not very great. Williams found that older doctors were more likely to make home visits but this is not always the case and was not so in Aberdeen.[25]

The age of the patient is a much more important factor than the age of the doctor in determining workload. Most studies show high consultation rates for the very young and the very old. Fry, Morrell and Hodgkin all found that these age groups had the highest proportion of patients consulting and also had the highest number of consultations per patient.[6,17,26]

There is also a close relationship between the age of the patient and the ratio of surgery attendances to home visits. In south-west England Wright found that the over 65s received as many home visits as they had surgery consultations.[8] Hopkins *et al* found that the visiting rate for the over 65s was four times as great as that for the under 65s and that although only 14 per cent of the patients in the practice were in the older age group, over half of his return visits were to them.[15] Even Morrell in central London, with his very high A/V ratio of ten attendances to one home visit, found that the ratio was less than two to one for the over 75s.[17]

Sex of Patients

Remarkably constant throughout the surveys is the finding that females create a greater workload than males. Morrell found that females consulted more frequently in every age group except 0-5, with an average rate of five times per year compared with four for males.[17] Eighty per cent of the females on his list consulted the doctor during the year, compared with 75 per cent of males.

Bebbington, a student who reported on a North Wales practice in a sheep farming area in 1969, found that 60 per cent of all consultations were by females.[27] Males predominated however in the age groups 11-20 and over 70. Cartwright also reported more consultations by females except in the 55-64 age group where there were almost equal numbers for each sex.

As would be expected all surveys show a heavy use of general practitioners by women in the 15-44 age group because of pregnancy and childbirth. In this respect the quite sharp decline in the number of births since 1966 will have been another factor reducing the doctor's workload. Wamoscher and Hull found that the higher consultation rate for females spread over all age groups.[28,29]

Mining practices are an exception. Rider *et al* (1969) found that both males and females had an average rate of six consultations per year, which was attributed to the very high consultation rate for males between the ages of 45 and 64.[10] Forty-one per cent of the men working in the district were employed in mining or quarrying.

Social Class

Whereas the findings regarding the age and sex of the patient are fairly conclusive there are conflicting statistics and differing conclusions concerning the extent to which social class affects workload. Inconsistent definitions of terms such as 'usage' and 'social class' are partly responsible, but differences in morbidity in different social classes also make the task of the researcher difficult.

Scot and McVie (1962) reported that social classes I and II were more likely than the other social classes to call the doctor for a home visit.[30] They also noted a higher follow-up rate of home visits for the higher social classes but patients in lower social classes asked for more late-night and evening calls.

Kedward reported in the same year on his three months' study of a rural practice on the edge of a coalfield.[31] He found that the proportion of households which consulted the doctor was least for the higher social classes and that they tended to avoid surgery consultations, relying on home visits and telephone calls.

Cartwright, from her analysis of patients' replies which was not subject to doctor's bias, found little difference in the consultation rate of middle-class and working-class patients over 45 years of age. Below 45 however she found that more working-class than middle-class patients under 45 consulted the doctor, and that 23 per cent of social classes III-V consulted over five times per year compared with 14 per cent of classes I-II. Picken and Ireland, (1969), analysing consultations in a village near Edinburgh, attributed the relatively high proportion of consultations with children from classes I and II to the higher degree of parental concern in those classes rather than to illness.[32] Morrell found that the highest consultation rate in his London practice was with social class III and the lowest with social class II.[17] Social class II had the highest ratio of surgery attendances to home visits and social class I had the lowest.

In contrast, Marsh *et al* found in their analysis of home visits in north-east England that social class V required twice the amount of visiting as might be expected from the proportion of patients in this class while social class III required proportionately fewer.[14] However, social class I received the highest proportion of follow-up visits, the proportion declining with the social class scale. The doctors in the practices studied thought that a higher proportion of social class I patients could have come to the surgery and that this proportion declined through the social scale. Patients in class V received more late-night and evening calls.

Other Causes

There is a general impression among doctors that patients newly arrived in an area are likely to use their general practitioners more than average and Whitfield (1972) has shown this statistically.[33]

Research has also substantiated the impression of many general practitioners that a small proportion of their patients cause a large proportion of their work. Manning (1967)[34] and Dinwoodie (1969)[35] found that 6 and 7 per cent of their patients caused between 20 and 25 per cent of their work, respectively.[34, 35] Wamoscher (1966) found that 15 per cent of his patients generated nearly 50 per cent of his total number of doctor contracts.[28]

Another factor which influences the doctor's workload is the season of the year. Most doctors take holidays during the summer with the result that their work during that period is taken over by their colleagues. This results in the difference in workload for the doctor between winter and summer being less than might be expected. Nevertheless there is a seasonal variation with the lowest workload in the summer months. Posner (1965) found August the quietest month, a gradual rise through the autumn, a pre-Christmas decline and the greatest workload from January to April.[9] Morrell found that the maximum consultation rate occurred between November and January.[17] McKnight and Jackson (1969) reported the usual easier pace in the summer with January and May as the heaviest months.[36] Wright found a high consultation rate in March and fewer consultations in December than in June.[8] Williams did not find any great seasonal variations in the doctor's workload.

Workload varies not only by season but also according to the days of the week. Most practices find Monday the busiest day. Eimerl and Pearson reported that Merseyside doctors had twice as many consultations on Mondays as on any other day.[37] Posner saw an average of 69 patients on Mondays, compared with his lightest day, Thursday, when he saw 28.[9] Marsh *et al* (1972) found that 28 per cent of new visits were requested on a Monday and that doctors did 23 per cent of repeat visits on a Monday also.[14]

There is one more self-evident factor which affects workload. Major epidemics of influenza distort the figures considerably. The heavy workload of the doctor is recognised by the Department of Health and Social Security which permits doctors, at such times, to issue certificates of inability to work to patients whom they have not seen.

Notes

1. A general practice glossary, 2nd edition (1973). *Jnl. R.C.G.P.*, Supplement No. 3, Vol 23.
2. Logan, W.P.D. and Cushion, A.A. (1958) *General Register Office Studies on Medical and Population Subjects. No 14, Morbidity Statistics from General Practitioners.* HMSO, London.
3. Cartwright, A. (1967) *Patients and their Doctors.* Routledge and Kegan Paul, London.
4. *Seventh Report of the Review Body* (1966). HMSO, London.
5. *The General Household Survey, Introductory Report* (1973). HMSO, London.
6. Royal College of General Practitioners (1970) *Present State and Future Needs of General Practice.* Reports from General Practice, No.XIII, 1970.

7. Royal College of General Practitioners (1970). *A study of general practitioners' workload in South Wales, 1965-66.* Reports from general practice, No XII, 1970.
8. Royal College of General Practitioners (1968) *General practice in south west England.* Reports from general practice, No .VIII, 1968.
9. Posner, B.H. (1965) The pattern of work in an industrial practice. *The Practitioner,* 1965, 195, 799-803.
10. Rider, J.G. *et al* (1969) A study of workload in a mining area practice. *Jnl. R.C.G.P.,* 1969, 17, 361-9.
11. Irvine, D. (1972) *Teaching practices, Royal College of General Practitioners, Report from General Practice,* 1972.
12. Brown, W. (1973) Personal communication, Easington Colliery, Durham.
13. Jackson, M.P. (1974) *The Price of Coal.* Croom Helm, London.
14. Marsh, G.N. *et al* (1972) Survey of home visiting by general practitioners in north-east England. *Brit. Med. J.* 1972, 1, 487-92.
15. Hopkins, E.J. *et al* (1968) The relation of patient's age, sex and distance from surgery to the demand on the family doctor. *Jnl. R.C.G.P.,* 1968, 16, 368-78.
16. Longmore, H.J.A. (1967) Description of Scottish rural practice, 1965. *Jnl. R.C.G.P.,* 1967, 13, 70-4.
17. Morrell, D.C. *et al* (1970) Patterns of demand in general practice, *Jnl. R.C.G.P.,* 1970, 19, 331-42.
18. Marsh, G.N. (1968) Visiting – falling workload in general practice. *Brit. Med. J.,* 1968, 1, 633-5.
19. Richardson, I.M. *et al* (1968) Patients geography in general practice. Attachment areas of Aberdeen practices. *Lancet,* 1968, ii, 1290-3.
20. Smith, F. and Seddon, T.M. (1968) Transport of patients in general practice. *Jnl. R.C.G.P.,* 1968, 15, 52-8.
21. Binnie, G.A.C. (1970) The possible effects of transport on a rural practice: a retrospective survey. *Jnl. R.C.G.P.,* 1970, 19, 143-5.
22. Lance, H. (1971) Report on transport services in general practice. An experiment in five general practices. *Jnl. R.C.G.P.,* 1971, 21 Supp. No. 3.
23. Department of Health and Social Security (1973) *Health and Personal Social Services Statistics for England.* HMSO, London.
24. Wintersgill, W. (1973) Recruitment of unrestricted principals in general practice. *Health Trends,* 5, 2, 26-7.
25. Richardson, I.M. *et al* (1973) A study of general practitioners' consultations in north-east Scotland. *Jnl. R.C.G.P.,* 1973, 23, 132-42.
26. Hodgkin, K. (1973) *Towards Earlier Diagnosis.* Churchill Livingstone, Edinburgh and London.
27. Bebbington, R. (1969) A review of 508 consecutive patients seen in general practice. *Jnl. R.C.G.P.,* 1969, 18, 27-37.
28. Wamoscher, Z. (1966) The returning patients. A survey of patients with high attendance rates. *Jnl. Coll. Gen. Pract.,* 1966, 11, 166.
29. Hull, F.M. (1969) Social class consultation patterns in rural general practice.*Jnl. R.C.G.P.,* 1969, 18, 65-71.
30. Scott, R. and McVie, D.H. (1962) Doctor in the house. *Jnl. R.C.G.P.,* 1962, 5, 72-85.
31. Kedward, H.N. (1962) Social class habits of consulting. *Brit. J. Prev. Soc. Med.,* 1962, 16, 147-52.
32. Picken, B. and Ireland, G. (1969) Family patterns of medical care utilisation. Possible influence of family size, role and social class, on illness behaviour. *J. Chron. Dis.,* 1969, 22, 181-91.
33. Whitfield, M.J. (1972) Relationship between year of registration and mobility. *Jnl. R.C.G.P.,* 22 , 675-8.
34. Manning, A.D., (1967) Workload in general practice. *Jnl. R.C.G.P.,* 1967,

14, 336-43.

35. Dinwoodie, H.P. (1969) An elementary use of a computer for morbidity recording in general practice. *Health Bull.*, 1969, 27, 6-14.
36. McKnight, S.G. and Jackson, W.E. (1969) Workload and morbidity in an urban general practice in 1967. *Ulster Med. J.*, 1969, 38, 47-50.
37. Eimerl, T.S. and Pearson, R.J.C. (1966) Working time in general practice: how general practitioners use their time. *Brit. Med. J.*, 1966, 2, 1549-54.

3. THE PRIMARY HEALTH CARE TEAM

Nursing Staff

In addition to the numerous factors discussed in the previous chapter, the general practitioner's workload is increasingly being altered by the work of the Primary Health Care Team. Patients, doctors, nurses, health visitors and midwives have all been affected by the attachment schemes which have come into operation over the last decade but many doctors have viewed these changes with suspicion. The Report on Integrated Health Services (1971) published in Scotland rightly observed that 'further progress in the realignment of practice work by delegation can only be achieved if general practitioners themselves are prepared to reconsider traditional assumptions about their role'.[1] However, it is now fairly generally accepted that non-medical professional staff have an important role to play in modern general practice. It is, therefore, relevant to discuss the nature of the work undertaken by such staff and the direction in which the development of the Primary Health Care Team is moving.

Hockey (1966) painted a dismal picture of the role of district nurses prior to attachment schemes.[2] She found that almost half of them never met a doctor and that another two fifths saw a doctor on average only once a month. Their work was restricted to home visits which they undertook at a rate of eleven or twelve a day. Three quarters of these visits were to patients over 65 years of age. All district nurses were state registered but much of their work could have been done equally well by the less highly qualified state enrolled nurses. There is an implicit criticism throughout Hockey's book of the low utilisation of the skills of a highly trained professional worker and the resultant poor job satisfaction.

Many studies have described the work undertaken by state registered nurses in practices.[3-19] These accouns show clearly that much of this work, including injections, dressings, chaperoning, testing urine and taking blood pressures, could be done by state enrolled nurses. Other nursing tasks such as immunisation and venepuncture could be done by these nurses if they were to receive some additional training. It is significant that in many of the doctors' reports, state registered and state enrolled nurses appear to work together without any job demarcation.

The need to differentiate the work suitable for nurses with different skills has been recognised. Warin considered the possibility of an hierarchical structure for the attached nursing team with a sister in charge.[20] At that time he considered this feasible only in very large practices working in health centres. However, many recent planning documents envisage an increasingly important role for the state enrolled nurse. The Joint Working Party for Attachment Nursing Services[21] foresaw a place for state enrolled nurses, nursing auxiliaries and bath attendants in supplying help for patients whose needs have only recently been appreciated. The Standing Nursing Advisory Committee's report on the State Enrolled Nurse (1971)[22] recommended that increasing use should be made of these nurses in local authority nursing services. The Standing Medical Advisory Committee recommended (1971)[23] that state enrolled nurses should become members of the group practice team and both the BMA Report on Primary Health Care Teams (1974) and the monograph *The Work of the Nursing Team in General Practice* (1974) emphasise delegation of work to its appropriate level in the nursing teams.[23, 24, 19]

Buckoke and Irvine (1971), in a provocative and farsighted review, proposed that the state enrolled nurse should undertake almost the entire range of the traditional domiciliary nursing tasks previously reserved for the state registered nurse.[25] They considered that the state enrolled nurse could also perform many of the routine nursing duties at the surgery which were normally undertaken by the doctor or state registered nurse. Furthermore, they suggested that this realignment of nursing tasks would enable the state enrolled nurse in her turn to be relieved of such routine duties as bathing the elderly and the infirm, helping patients in and out of bed and dressing and undressing them.

If so much work which is traditionally performed by the state registered nurse can be delegated to her less well qualified colleague, what use can be made of her special skills outside the hospital service? It is evident that as a senior member of the Primary Health Care Team her role will be more supervisory but she will still continue to perform some technical tasks. Her most important one will be to take over work which is currently being done by the doctor. Once this happens the saving in time and effort for him will be considerable. As has been suggested, even the state enrolled nurse can undertake many tasks which have formerly been done almost exclusively by the doctor.

In 1967, Weston Smith and Mottram shook traditional general practice by describing a scheme in which a nurse made first home visits in place of the doctor.[26] The nurse answered telephone requests for home visits and went to see the patient herself if she thought she could cope with the situation or if she had any doubt about the need for a visit by the doctor. Weston Smith and Mottram believed that a state registered nurse with at least four years' experience after registration was competent to assess whether patients were ill enough to need a visit from the doctor. Their nurse paid 785 visits of which 485 were to patients aged 0-10, 133 to patients over 65 and 167 to patients aged 10-65. Only 10 per cent of the children to whom she made a first visit had to be visited by the doctor later in the day. The doctors found that this arrangement was acceptable to the majority of the patients. They considered three conditions essential for the operation of such a scheme; the doctors have to satisfy themselves that the nurses are capable of such work, the nurses must make a written report on each visit and discuss the treatment with the doctor, and the nurses undertaking this work have to receive special training probably within a general practice setting. Weston Smith and Mottram also described the use of nurses for monitoring the progress of acutely ill patients who had already been seen by the doctor at home, and for sharing with the doctor routine visits to the chronic elderly and chronic housebound sick. This was less controversial but still not generally accepted. A later paper from the same practice described the use of nurses for visiting patients who had been discharged from hospital, and for technical procedures such as venepunctures.[27]

Other doctors experimented with nurse visiting schemes at about the same time. Marsh (1969) analysed the work of a nurse which included visiting patients who had asked for a visit from the doctor.[15] Hasler *et al* (1968), in a similar study, identified the role of their nurses as similar to that of a hospital ward sister.[11] They agreed with Weston Smith and Mottram that nurses undertaking home visits should receive special training.

The Royal College of General Practitioners and the Department of Health and Social Security jointly produced a monograph called *The Practice Nurse* (1968).[10] This carefully evaluated study from official and authoritative sources gave the seal of respectability to the nurse's new role. For the first time, an estimate was made of the amount of doctor's time which a practice nurse could save. A nurse working for two and a half to three and a half hours per 1,000 patients per week was thought to be able to reduce the doctor's working hours by between 4 and 6 per cent.

Kuenssberg, who recorded the workload in his large Edinburgh group practice for well over twelve years, was convinced that the practice nurse saved the doctor much time and effort. In his James McKenzie lecture to the Royal College of General Practitioners in 1971, he emphasised that the employment of nurses in his practice had resulted in more thorough clinical medicine.[28] The time available for history taking had increased by 14 per cent, the use of diagnostic instruments and of rectal and pelvic examinations had increased by almost one half, the proportion of specimens sent to the laboratory had risen by nearly a third and the referral of patients to hospital had diminished appreciably. Despite this more thorough clinical medicine, the doctor's total workload in terms of hours had decreased by about 2 per cent. This time-saving was achieved by transferring a large proportion of home visits to the nurse including selected first visits which he termed assessment visits. One hundred patients who received such visits were asked their opinion about them and maintained that they were satisfied with them. Kuenssberg (1969) completely reorganised his nursing staff following local authority attachment of district nurses.[29] In the month in which his study took place a thousand traditional doctor-patient contacts were undertaken by nurses. Amongst these were 616 first contacts for minor illnesses such as cuts, boils and chicken pox and 319 follow-up visits by the nurse to patients who had first been seen by the doctor.

Other doctors have reported favourably on their experience in cooperating with their nursing staff. Rowland *et al* (1970), reviewing the Bristol attachment scheme, commented on the increase of about one third in the number of patients referred by general practitioners for home nursing after the commencement of the scheme.[16] He thought that this extra work fulfilled a previously unmet need as well as relieving the doctor of tasks which were more appropriate for a nurse. Moore *et al* (1973) found that a nurse, completely untrained and inexperienced in general practice, was able to decide what action to take when carrying out new visits to patients at home quite as accurately as the general practitioner.[30] She could competently decide whether to reassure the patient, send him to the next surgery or call the doctor. One fifth merely required reassurance and almost a half could attend the surgery. The significance of this finding is somewhat reduced since it refers to urban Scottish patients who are known to generate a high visiting rate.[31]

Most doctors who have written on this topic support the principle of district nurses undertaking a small proportion of new visits if the nurses have had appropriate training and experience and have good communications with the doctor. The Report on the Integrated Health Service (1971) was enthusiastic in recommending the use of nurses for first visits because of the success which had been achieved where this had been done 'with careful attention to preparation and a clear definition of the limits of nurses' discretion'.[1] Nevertheless this development is still questioned. Eight of the nine members of the Joint Working Party on the Attachment of Nursing Services to General Practice (1970) supported first visits by nurses.[21] However, one member, a midwife, felt so strongly on the subject that she wrote a note of reservation which ended: 'This is not a duty for which these members of the local authority staff are at present trained.' Perhaps her reservation might not have been made if appropriate training had been available.

The Standing Medical Advisory Committee (1971) saw considerable potential for the development of work in which the 'nurse acts on behalf of a doctor in situations which call for a decision'.[23] The committee stressed however that the nurse must not become a barrier between doctor and patient and that she should receive specific training if she is to assume these new functions.

The Briggs Report (1972) was rather more guarded.[32] It conceded that 'the infiltration of nurses and midwives into the diagnostic and therapeutic sphere is not necessarily harmful to the patient if medical supervision is good'. In a later passage, it refers to first visits by nurses attached to group practices as the area which requires the most thorough and continuing discussion between the two professions. The Report of the Board of Science and Education (BMA 1974) was adamant in stating that state registered nurses should be used effectively and with a full recognition of their skills.[24] It supported the Briggs report in believing that the training of nurses should involve considerable experience of community nursing and that implementation of this policy was long overdue. In order to convince the more wary members of the medical establishment that nurses can be used more effectively in practices, the report suggests that a controlled experiment should be set up to compare practices in which nurses share decision-making responsibilities with those in which they do not.

Appropriate training appears to be the key which will open up new areas of work and responsibility for the state registered nurse working in the community. A start in this direction has already been made. Hodes (1972) described a teaching programme for nurses and health visitors which had been developed over a three-year period in an eight-man group practice in Hertfordshire.[33] Hasler *et al* (1972) described an extended day release course for both general practice nurses and local authority nurses in the Thames Valley area.[34] This course centred on the surgery work of the nurse. The failure of a panel established by the Joint Board of Clinical Nursing Studies (1974) to devise a syllabus of training for the nurse in the Primary Health Care Team resulted in strong letters of protest from both the Royal College of Nursing and the Royal College of General Practitioners.[35,36,37] Accordingly the joint board is setting up another panel whose members will have a greater commitment to its success.[38] The state registered nurse's new role in the community now seems well on the way to being established. The state enrolled nurse needs to be trained and prepared to take over many of the tasks which were traditionally assigned to her state registered colleague.

Forman (1974) surveyed nurse attachments in south-west England.[39] Although providing a proportion of useful criticism over 90 per cent of practices felt that district nurse attachment had improved the service to the patient.

Health Visitors

There is a considerable variation throughout England and Wales in the number of health visitors who are members of Primary Health Care Teams. General practitioners had little prior understanding of the work of health visitors who traditionally have been more independent than district nurses. Some of the health visitors' work had been taken over by the doctors and the practice nurses before attachment schemes had been arranged. This has contributed to health visitors having a less well defined role in the Primary Health Care Team than nurses and less impact on the doctor's workload.

The National Health Service Act 1946 laid down that health visitors were to 'give advice as to the care of young children, to expectant and nursing mothers, to persons suffering from illness and to take such measures as would prevent the spread of infection'.[40] Much of this work is now being done by other members of the Primary Health Care Team. State enrolled nurses run immunisation sessions, state registered nurses make follow-up visits to sick children, and social workers and marriage guidance counsellors give support to problem families, unmarried mothers and couples having matrimonial problems. The role of the health visitor seems destined to change.

Studies of health visitors working as members of Primary Health Care Teams show that their traditional role can be extended and the distinctive nature of their work acknowledged.[41-50] Ante-natal care involving advice on mothercraft, breast feeding, relaxation exercises and the organisation of classes for fathers is an area of work for which they are well equipped by experience and training. They also have a statutory duty to visit young children soon after they are born. They can organise immunisation schemes and be responsible for their success. Their liaison with the school health service supports their role as health educators. In some practices, health visitors have been concerned with the care of the elderly. This leads to a greater recognition of the unmet clinical and social needs of these patients. In the short term this may increase the general practitioner's workload but as some of the health visitor's work with the elderly is preventive, it may lessen the doctor's workload in the long term.

Many reports indicate that health visitors are still most active in the ante-natal and pediatric field; it is probable that they will find their most distinctive role in the development of this work. The monitoring of the development and progress of children has now become a recognised function of medicine. This could lead to a considerable increase in the doctor's workload but it should be greatly lightened by close cooperation with a health visitor. Some practice pediatric record cards already contain space for the clinical notes which health visitors make at well-baby clinics, together with percentile graphs of length, weight and head circumference. The doctor need only carry out the important comprehensive physical examination of the child a few days after birth and again at the age of six weeks.

The main effect of the attachment of health visitors to group practices appears to be an extension of the work undertaken by the practice rather than a lessening of the doctor's workload. Ambler *et al* (1968), in a study of three county boroughs in England and Wales, found that of fifty doctors who had a health visitor in their practice, thirteen thought that their work had increased in some areas and decreased in others, twenty-two thought their own workload had diminished and three thought it had increased, while twelve either noticed no change or did not know how they had been affected.[42]

Allen and King (1968) concluded that the range and amount of the health visitor's work increased after attachment and the improved communication between doctor and health visitor encouraged the referral of patients between the two professions.[43] No assessment was made of work saved but the overall impression was that everybody's workload increased. Fry *et al* (1965) however thought that the health visitor reduced the doctor's workload, especially in polio immunisation, cooperation with the social services and the management of infant care problems.[41] Warin (1968) did not find that the discovery of unmet social needs increased the doctors' work as health visitors either dealt with the problems themselves or contacted the appropriate social service agency.[20]

Midwives

Midwife attachment schemes are least well documented. As a result there is no clear analysis of the midwife's work and of the amount of time and effort saved for the doctor. There are two distinct views on the future role of the midwife. Buckoke and Irvine (1971) see her function restricted to the hospital; they regard the clinical responsibility during the ante and post-natal periods as primarily belonging to the doctor and suggest that he should be assisted in this by the health visitor while the state enrolled nurse should attend to the practical nursing procedures.[25] However, a strong case can be made for giving the midwife more work and more responsibility in the ante-natal and puerperal period. She could replace the doctor in routine ante-natal care, referring to him only deviations from the norm. In Britain this system has been widely practised during labour for many years and a similar one might operate equally well in the ante-natal and puerperal periods.

At the majority of deliveries, no doctor is present and if there are no complications the midwife produces excellent results. Butler and Bonham's perinatal mortality survey (1963) showed clearly that babies whose mothers consulted only a midwife throughout their pregnancy had the lowest mortality rate.[51] This appears to indicate the ability of midwives to recognise abnormalities and refer them to the doctor. The survey also showed good results when the care of the patient was shared between the general practitioner and the midwife.

Care during labour has always been the core of the midwife's work. Increasing the proportion of hospital deliveries to over 90 per cent has meant that the district midwife has been in danger of losing her distinctive role.[52] However, in some areas the obstetric work of the midwife and the general practitioner has not decreased as much as was anticipated. Very early discharge schemes were pioneered in Salford where the district midwife admitted her patients to a hospital unit, delivered them and discharged them home to her own care.[52] Such schemes have proliferated. The most likely development however is that district midwives will be absorbed into the hospital service and that all deliveries will take place in hospital. If this happens it is to be hoped that midwives will continue to provide some care for their patients outside the hospital and that they will be attached to group practices to provide ante-natal and puerperal care. This would ensure that their status within the community is maintained and that they continue to share the responsibility for their patients with the general practitioner, thus reducing his workload.

Social Workers

The Seebohm Committee on Local Authority and Allied Personal Social Services (1968) considered that 'doctors have been slow in coming to terms with the new social work "helping profession" that is growing so rapidly alongside them'.[53] It claimed that 'doctors are ill trained themselves to deal with the psychological and social factors in the management of illness and the prevention of chronic disability and dependency; nor do they know how to get help from social agencies and to collaborate with social workers – who have *their* contribution to make and a professional responsibility to do so'. It was hesitant about recommending attachment of social workers to health centres as 'unfortunately there is no evidence that general practice is as yet ready for such a programme'. The report did however acknowledge that 'general practice today is in touch with a higher proportion of those who are in difficulties than any other of the social services and it needs the full support of them all' and in its conclusion recommended that 'as soon as doctors ... feel they want a worker of the social service department to be "attached" to them to become a member also of *their* team, the department should do all it can to meet their request'. Indeed Jefferys had remarked several years earlier that 33 per cent of all the patients seen by general practitioners in an unselected series of consultations were known by the doctor to have socio-economic as well as medical problems thought to be relevant to their symptoms.[54]

The BMA Report on Primary Health Care Teams (1974) states emphatically that 'the social aspects of medical care fall essentially within the function of the Primary Health Care Team and the social worker should, therefore, be a part of that organisation.[24] In any subsequent reorganisation of health and social services this situation should be recognised'.

At a practical level the Department of Health and Social Security Report on Social Work Support for the Health Services (1974) recommends that all health centres should have accommodation for social workers.[55]

As yet, little is known about the effect which attaching a social worker might have on the workload of the doctor. If the social services were able to provide adequate community care, the task of the doctor would certainly be easier. Higher standards of nutrition, warmth, housing, nurseries, special schools, sheltered accommodation and hostels for the most vulnerable members of the community would improve their health and well-being. Formal links between doctors and social workers will facilitate the referral of clients between these two professions; also, there is scope for links between the Primary Health Care Team and churches, marriage guidance councils and various voluntary aid groups.[56] If effective help is given to those in need, their apparent 'medical' needs would diminish. In such a setting, it will be necessary for general practitioners to consider carefully whether their patients' illnesses are essentially 'social' and could thus be more effectively dealt with by social workers who are trained and qualified to deal with such problems. The BMA Report on Primary Health Care Teams (1974) recommended that there should be a basic generalist social work training which would enable social workers to be fully integrated into teams, while those with additional specialist training, in child care or mental disorder for example, should be available for consultation.[24]

There have been some studies of the extent to which doctors have referred patients to social workers. At the Caversham Centre in London the referral rate was about 25 per 1,000 patients per year after the initial backlog of cases was resolved. Wolfe and Teed (1967) reported that in Saskatoon 6 general practitioners working in one centre referred on average 25 patients per year.[58] Ratoff (1970) in Liverpool had a referral rate of 26 per 1,000.[59] In the Derby social work attachment scheme (1971), the 67 participating doctors each referred, on average, 14 patients per year.[60] Forman (1968) reported an average referral rate of 10 per 1,000 for his practice but noted the great variation in the degree of cooperation with social workers by individual partners.[61]

In most of these schemes, the workload passing from the doctor to the social worker appears to have been small. This may be partly because social workers are already aware of many of the social problems in an area and that the formal links between social workers and doctor are helpful mostly in an informative way, enabling each worker to know the aims, objects and methods of the other. It may also be due to attachments taking place mostly in areas where good informal links have already been established. On the other hand Ratoff (1973) considered general practitioners far too conservative as well as being ignorant of the social workers role.[62] He considered that relationships were poor and that face-to-face contact was the all-important remedy.[63]

It is reasonable to suppose that the potential scope for referral is substantially greater. At present, social service departments in most parts of the country suffer from a rapid staff turnover, are woefully short of professionally qualified social workers and have inadequate resources to meet the demands made upon them. Contrary to the view expressed by the Seebohm Committee it is probable that social workers rather than general practitioners are not yet ready for attachment schemes.

Notes

1. Scottish Home and Health Department (1972) *Report of a Working Group: The Nurses in an Integrated Health Service.* HMSO, London.
2. Hockey, L. (1966) *Feeling the Pulse: a study of district nursing in six areas.* Queen's Institute of District Nursing, London.
3. Sanctuary, J.C.T. *et al* (1965) Anciliary help in general practice. *Jnl. R.C.G.P.,* 1965, 9, 55-63.
4. Marsh, G.N. (1967) Group practice nurse: an analysis and comment on six months' work. *Brit. Med. J.,* 1967, i, 489-91.
5. Baldwin, J.T. (1967) The use of the nurse in general practice. *Jnl. Coll. Gen. Pract.,* 1967, 13, 364-7.
6. Hodgkin, G.K.H. (1967) Saving doctor's time with a practice nurse. Conference: The Team. *Family Health Care,* 1967.
7. Murray, J. (1967) Fifteen years in general practice. *Jnl. R.C.G.P.,*1967, 13, 367-72.
8. Gray, L.J. (1967) The Team, signpost to the future. *Family Health Care.* 1967.
9. Hasler, J.C. *et al* (1968) Development of the nursing section of the community health team. *Brit. Med. J.,* 1968, 3, 734-6.
10. Royal College of General Practitioners (1968) *The Practice Nurse.* Reports from General Practice, No.10, 1968.
11. Hasler, J.C. and Stewart, T.I. (1969) The consultation in general practice. *Jnl. R.C.G.P.,* 1969, 16, 31-8.
12. Dixon P.N. (1969) Work of a nurse in a health centre treatment room. *Brit. Med. J.,* 1969, 4, 292-4.
13. Dixon, P.N. and Trounson, E. (1969) Evaluation of health centre community nurse team. *Brit. Med. J.,* 1969, 1, 306-9.
14. Hunter, D.A. (1969) Doctors and nurses in Brent. A study in group attachment. *Nursing Times,* 1969, 65, 560-2.
15. Marsh, G.N. (1969) Visiting nurse – analysis of one year's work. *Brit. Med. J.,* 1969, 4, 42-4.
16. Rowland, A.J. *et al* (1970) Evaluation of home nurse attachment in Bristol. *Brit. Med. J.,* 1970, 4, 545-7.
17. Howard, A.L. (1970) Twelve months' attachment: from the local authority. *Nursing Times,* 1970, 66, 1390-1.

18. Hockey, L. and Buttimore, A (1970) Cooperation in patient care. Q.I.D.N.
19. Gilmore, M. *et al* (1974) *The work of the nursing team in general practice.* Council for the Education and Training of Health Visitors.
20. Warin, J.F. (1968) General practitioners and nursing staff: a complete attachment scheme in retrospect and prospect. *Brit. Med. J.*, 1968, 2, 41-5.
21. Department of Health and Social Security (1970) *Report of Joint Working Party on Group Attachment. Attachment of Nursing Services to General Practice.* HMSO, London.
22. Central Health Services Council (1971) *Standing Nursing Advisory Committee Report on the State Enrolled Nurse.* HMSO, London.
23. Department of Health and Social Security Welsh Office (1971) *Organisation of Group Practice.* A report of the Sub-Committee of the Standing Medical Advisory Committee. HMSO, London.
24. British Medical Association (1974) Board of Science and Education: *Primary Health Care Teams.*
25. Buckoke, Y.E. and Irvine, D. (1971) Nursing in the community; a time for reform? *Nursing Times,* 1971, 133-6.
26. Weston Smith, J. and Mottram, E.M. (1967) Extended use of nursing services in general practice. *Brit. Med. J.*, 1967, 4, 672-4.
27. Weston Smith, J. and Donovan, J.B. (1970) The practice nurse – new look. *Brit. Med. J.*, 1970, 4, 637-77.
28. Kuenssberg, E.V. (1971) General practice through the looking glass (the James McKenzie lecture). *The Practitioner,* 1971, 206, 129-45.
29. Kuenssberg, E.V. (1970) Suppl. No.3, Vol.19, *Jnl. R.C.G.P.*, 1970.
30. Moore, M.S. *et al* (1973) First contact decisions in general practice. *Lancet,* 1973, 1, 817-19.
31. Stevenson, J.S.K. (1964) General practice in Scotland – why the differences? *Brit. Med. J.*, 1, 1370-3.
32. Department of Health and Social Security (1972) *Report of the Committee on Nursing (Briggs Report). HMSO, London.*
33. Hodes, C. (1972) Education of nurses and health visitors in group practice. *Jnl. R.C.G.P.*, 1972, 22, 477.
34. Hasler, J.C. *et al* (1972) Training for the treatment room sister in general practice. *Brit. Med. J.*, 1972, 1, 232-4.
35. Minutes of Meeting of Joint Board of Clinical Nursing Studies, 2 October 1974 (Not published).
36. Letter from Royal College of Nursing to Joint Board of Clinical Nursing Studies, 14 January 1975 (Not published).
37. Letter from Royal College of General Practitioners to Joint Board of Clinical Nursing Studies, January 1975 (Not published).
38. Minutes of meeting of Joint Board of Clinical Nursing Studies, 9 April 1975 (Not published).
39. Forman, J.A.S. (1974) Nurse attachment to general practice in south-west England. *Jnl. R.C.G.P.*, 1974, 24, 579-81.
40. *National Health Service Act* (1946). HMSO, London.
41. Fry, J. *et al* (1965) The evolution of a health team: a successful general practitioner-health visitor attachment. *Brit. Med. J.*, 1965, 1, 181-3.
42. Ambler, M. *et al* (1968) The attachment of local health authority staff to general practice. *Med. officer,* 119, 295-9.
43. Allen W.H. and King, V.M. (1968) A study of health visitor attachments to general practitioners in Hertfordshire. *Med. Officer,*

1968, 119, 177-80.
44. Lewis, T.D. (1968) Health visitor and the family doctor. *Jnl. R.C.G.P.*, 1968, 15, 241-3.
45. Parish, P.A. (1968) Health visitor attachment in general practice. *Nursing Times,* 1968, 64, 256-9.
46. Player, D.A. (1969) Attachment of health visitors and district nurses and midwives to general practice in Dumfries. *Update,* 1969, 1, 641-5.
47. Jobling, D. (1969) The work of an 'attached' health visitor. *Brit. J. Med. Educ.* 1969.
48. Williamson, J. *et al* (1966) The use of health visitors in preventative geriatrics. *Geront. Clin.*, 1966, 8, 362-9.
49. Ness, M.T. and Reekie, M.M. (1970) Old people in a group practice. *Nursing Times,* 1970, 66, 1232-3.
50. Williams, E.I. *et al* (1972) Sociomedical study of patients over 75 in general practice. *Brit. Med. J.*, 1972, 2, 445-8.
51. Butler, N.R. and Bonham, D.G. (1963) *Perinatal Mortality.* E. & S. Livingstone, Edinburgh and London.
52. Rawlings, E.E. (1970) A general practitioner short stay delivery unit. *Practitioner,* 1970, 204, 825-30.
53. *Report of Committee on local authority and Allied Personal Social Services,* (Seebohm Report) (1968). HMSO, London.
54. Jefferys, M. (1965) *Anatomy of social welfare services.* Michael Joseph, London.
55. Department of Health and Social Security Welsh Office (1974) *Social Work Support for the Health Service.* HMSO, London.
56. Marsh, G.N. and Barr, J. (1975) Marriage guidance counselling in a group practice. *Jnl. R.C.G.P.*, 1975, 25, 73.
57. Goldberg, E.M. *et al* (1968) Social work in general practice. *Lancet,* 1968, 552-5.
58. Wolfe, S. and Teed, G. (1967) The study of the work of a medical social worker in group medical practice. *Canadian Medical Association Journal,* 96, 1407-16.
59. Ratoff, L. and Pearson, B. (1970) Social casework in general practice: an alternative approach. *Brit. Med. J.*, 1970, 2, 475-7.
60. Cooper, B. (1971) Social work in general practice: the Derby scheme. *Lancet,* 1971, 1, 539-42.
61. Forman, J.A.S. and Fairburn, E.M. (1968) *Social Casework in General Practice.* Oxford University Press, London.
62. Ratoff, L. (1973) More Social work for general practice. *Jnl. R.C.G.P.*, 1973, 23, 736.
63. Ratoff, L. *et al* (1974) Social workers and general practitioners – some problems of working together. *Jnl. R.C.G.P.*, 1974, 24, 750.

4 A PROFILE OF THE NORTON PRACTICE

The Environment

The chief aim of the survey undertaken in the Norton practice in 1972 was to analyse the workload created for one doctor and the other members of the Primary Health Care Team by the patients on his list. The area in which the practice is situated, the characteristics of the patients on the list, and the composition of the Primary Health Care Team, of which the doctor was a member are all factors which have to be considered before the findings on workload can be discussed and their significance evaluated.

The group practice centre is situated in Norton, a suburb of Stockton-on-Tees, a large town in Cleveland county in the industrial north-east of England. At one time it was a village and there are still reminders of the period before it was absorbed by the large town. A broad north to south High Street is flanked by a mixture of modern commercial premises and older residential property. At the north end there is an extensive village green with the traditional duck pond, parish church and school. Sixty-six per cent of the 15,000 patients registered with the group live in Norton itself, while the rest live in the neighbouring town of Billingham.

The Patients

The survey covered approximately 3,100 people, all of whom were on the list of one doctor in the practice at the beginning of 1972 or who registered with the doctor during that year (see Appendix I).

The age structure of the list of patients is not quite identical to that of England and Wales.[1] There is a larger proportion of school children of both sexes, a lower proportion of adults in the 45-64 age group and a slightly lower proportion of pre-school children. These variations are however not sufficient to affect the workload of the practice to any marked extent. The proportion of patients aged 65 and over is normal, an important fact as elderly people create a heavier workload than other patients.

Forty-nine per cent of the patients are male, a sex ratio which is almost the same as that for England and Wales at the 1971 population census.[1] As the sex of the patient causes differences in workload, this characteristic of the practice is important.

The list varies from the norm in its social class structure. The latest figures show that 20 per cent of households in England and Wales belong to social classes I and II and 29 per cent to classes IV and V.[1] The figures for the 1,482 households studied were 26 and

19 per cent respectively. The practice contains about 55 per cent of social class III households compared with the national average of 51 per cent. The evidence on the differing use of doctors according to social class is somewhat confused, but it seems highly unlikely that the small divergences from average in the social class structure of the practice could account for more than a marginal decrease or increase in workload.

There is not a great deal of evidence to substantiate the impression of many doctors that mobile patients cause more work than patients in stable communities.[2] Nevertheless, mobility was taken into account in analysing the characteristics of patients in this practice. Only about 25 per cent of patients had been on the list for over twenty years while 60 per cent had been on it for over ten years. The number of patients on the list has remained almost constant over the last ten years between 3 and 7 per cent joining or leaving the practice annually. There is no reason to suppose that the practice is unusual in this respect

Very few studies have been made of the distribution of patients' homes in relation to their doctors' premises. In this study it was found that about 25 per cent of patients lived within half a mile of the surgery, 33 per cent between a half and one mile, 33 per cent between one and two miles and the remaining 10 per cent over two miles. As has been mentioned earlier, 800 patients registered with the practice were transferred in 1966 to other doctors nearer to their homes as they lived so far from the surgery that they were creating a disproportionate amount of travelling time both for themselves and for the doctor. Exceptions were made for seriously or chronically ill patients and the very old. The comparatively compact practice in Norton is partly the result of this policy. The cross-section of patients appears to be fairly typical of English urban practices. None of the factors which have been considered suggest that the workload should be abnormally high or low. It is also necessary to consider whether the practice itself has any distinctive features which might affect workload.

Premises and Staff

The practice premises are about 150 years old. The exterior of the building is austere but behind this facade there is a bright and modern group practice centre. The interior of the building was substantially modified and extended in 1965 and 1970. Thirty per cent of the cost of the improvements was borne by the Department of Health and Social Security. The remainder of the capital was borrowed by the partners from the General Practice Finance Corporation.

The improved premises provide adequate facilities for both the doctors and the other members of the team, including a nurse's treatment room and a health visitor's office. The provision of a children's play area is one feature which makes the waiting time for patients as pleasant as possible. Secretarial and reception areas are well equipped with intercoms, dictaphones, electric calculators and other aids to efficiency.

The premises contain a side room in which many of the simpler diagnostic techniques are carried out by doctor or nurse. There are facilities for urinalysis, microscopic and chemical tests on urine and faeces, and for determining erythrocte sedimentation rates.

During the workload study the following staff were working in the practice:

(1) Five doctors and two trainee general practitioners.
For the last ten years the practice has had five doctors in partnership. It was recognised as a teaching practice under the Newcastle University training scheme in 1970. Two trainees are attached to the practice, each joining for a six-month period.

(2) Nursing and lay staff employed by the doctors include:
Two state registered nurses.
Three full-time receptionists.
One part-time (evening) receptionist.
Two filing clerks.
One administrative secretary.
One research secretary, supported by a grant from the regional hospital board.

(3) Staff attached from the local authority include:
One health visitor.
One midwife.
Two state registered nursing sisters (formerly district nurses).
One state enrolled nurse, shared with another practice.

(4) Community workers liaising with the practice on a regular, normally weekly basis include:
One qualified social worker.
The local Anglican vicar.
One marriage guidance counsellor.

It is the aim of the group practice centre to provide all the health requirements of patients but there are still some gaps in this comprehensive scheme. As yet, there is no family planning clinic and a few patients attend clinics in the area for contraceptive advice and cervical smear tests. Mothers and babies living more than pram-pushing distance from the medical centre sometimes attend local authority child welfare clinics for advice when these are more conveniently situated than the well-baby clinic at the centre. On average only two patients per week receive non-referred care from the two nearby hospital casualty departments, one of which is two miles and the other five miles from the surgery. Some patients use industrial medical centres in cases of minor illness but these patients are usually referred to their own doctor for illnesses which are at all serious and for certification of incapacity to work.

With his large supporting team, it is evident that the doctor's workload should be considerably less than it was in earlier years when he worked alone. The employment of two practice nurses by the doctors in addition to local authority nursing staff results in a total of eleven and a half hours of nursing care per 1,000 patients per week. The health visitor works for two and a half hours per 1,000 patients. Details of the workload of the doctor and of these workers will be given in the next chapter. An appropriate delegation of work by the doctor following a careful assessment of all relevant circumstances, and a willingness of patients to approach other team members direct, ensure that work is distributed amongst the team. In addition to the professional staff, the practice uses as many as eighteen hours of clerical time per 1,000 patients per week. This improves the administration of the practice and results in a more efficient use of professional time.

Method of Working

The administrative secretary is responsible for the administration of the practice and for all members of staff except those employed by the local authority. Her duties include financial matters, income tax, correspondence with the executive council, wages and duty rotas. She reports through a partner to a board meeting of the doctors which is held approximately every six weeks. She also liaises with the accountant, architect, solicitor, bank manager and other professional people and at times arranges their attendance at board meetings when relevant matters are discussed. The work of the practice in caring for patients is co-ordinated by doctors and other members of the team at informal daily meetings over morning coffee. The administrative secretary and community workers attend this meeting about once a week.

Various schemes for the improved care of patients have evolved from a lunch arranged by the practice approximately every two months. The partners entertain medical and non-medical guests and discuss problems of mutual interest regarding the community. A developmental pediatric programme, as well as closer liaison with social workers, the church and marriage guidance counsellors, have evolved from these meetings.

The practice has an established principle that, whenever possible, work should be undertaken by those best suited to it. Ideally, all members of the team should feel that they are doing work appropriate to their skills and training, and that they are not spending time on tasks which could be done by people less skilled than themselves. State registered nurses should not be doing simple dressings, nor should doctors be doing venepunctures; prophylactic immunization programmes, although planned and coordinated by health visitors, should be administered by nurses. Limitation of staff means that there must be flexibility in implementing this policy but the acknowledgement of policy objectives is an important first step.

There is a danger that the group practice system will depersonalise that branch of medicine which has most to gain from personal care. The delegation of work to the non-medical members of the team, the ready availability of partners to deputise during the doctor's absence and the use of remote deputising services all accentuate this danger. Strenuous efforts have been made in this practice to avoid depersonalisation.

Following a long-established tradition, each patient has been accustomed to looking upon one member of the group as his own doctor. Other doctors were only consulted in emergencies or when the patient's own doctor was not available. In 1971 the record system was changed and each partner had the records of his own patients filed separately. This enabled him to study them more readily, to have easier access to the cards and also simplified the filing procedure. This change has produced an interesting and important side-effect. Patients have to know who their doctor is in order that the receptionist can find the right record, which means that the personal doctor scheme has become formalised. By retaining one of the main virtues of the single-handed practice system, the group practice has been rescued from becoming efficient but impersonal. The doctor can give personal service to his patients and coordinate the other members of the team in their tasks. The responsibility, both moral and legal, for the care given by the team rests firmly and solely with the doctor.

The fact that patients are encouraged to rely more or less entirely on the services of their own doctor presents problems. It makes it essential that the doctor should make himself available to his patients at all times, except for certain regular and reasonable off-duty periods. The schedule (see page 52) shows the availability of one doctor in the group, the others having similar hours. Each partner is on duty one evening a week and for one weekend in every five from 10 a.m. on Saturdays to 8 a.m. on Mondays. Night calls (midnight until 8 a.m.) are carried out by each doctor for his own patients. Each doctor has six weeks' holiday and one week study leave a year. The patients' own doctor is available for approximately 50 per cent of the time, taking into account holidays, weekends and off-duty periods. Nevertheless, in the year studied, no less than 84 per cent of consultations by patients were with their own doctor, demonstrating that the personalised doctor system is practicable, even allowing for adequate time off for the doctor. A flexible appointment system which can accommodate urgent as well as routine consultations is however essential. An over-booked appointment system or a lengthy waiting period will militate against a personal doctor service.

It is possible that some patients might occasionally prefer to see a different doctor. In this practice, such patients are allowed to 'float'. Others, who lose confidence in their doctor or who have difficulty in establishing a satisfactory rapport, can change to a different doctor within the group by intimitating their wish to the receptionist and their chosen doctor. This is a very rare occurrence; only one family during the last three years has transferred from the list of the doctor whose practice is being studied.

Hospital Services

The workload of the practice and the standard of service it can provide must depend to some extent on the quality and availability of the hospital services in the area. This medical centre is fortunate in receiving strong support from the local hospitals. Acute emergencies can be admitted to hospital immediately, due to the proper functioning of a well-organised bed bureau. Two general casualty departments and one eye and ENT department are open day and night for emergency treatment and for minor surgical operations for patients referred to them. As is unfortunately often the case, the waiting lists for non-urgent cases for both out-patient attendance and in-patient treatment are often long, particularly in some specialities.

The obstetric facilities for general practitioners at the local district maternity hospital are extremely comprehensive. No babies are delivered at home but there is a very early discharge unit to which mothers who would formerly have had their babies at home are admitted. The district midwife and general practitioner are in attendance and the mother and baby can be discharged a few hours after delivery. General practitioners also have access to a ward of thirty beds where patients who are not expected to have any complications are delivered. Formal booking into this ward is for forty-eight hours or nine days but patients are discharged when appropriate. Abnormal obstetric cases are referred to specialist care in other wards of the hospital. The cooperation between the specialist obstetricians and the general practitioners is excellent.

A pathology collecting service calls at the surgery daily at 1 p.m. from Monday to Friday. This regular service facilitates patient investigations by transporting specimens to the laboratory and bringing back reports. The laboratory will carry out any test which the doctor requests and has recently extended the service to include virological investigations. Full use can be made of this service as a nurse is always available to take relevant specimens. Post-mortems of patients who died at home can also be arranged with the local pathologist.

The radiology department of the local hospital provides full X-ray facilities for general practitioners. No appointment is needed for chest X-rays, but it is necessary to make appointments for X-rays such as barium meals which need more elaborate techniques. Open access to such diagnostic facilities enhances the interest which the doctor obtains from his work and increases the care which he can provide for his patients. It also obviates the need for many referrals to out-patient departments for specialist opinion.

The group practice in Norton is a fully developed team practice with adequate premises. The doctors receive much support from other members of the team and are helped in the smooth running of the practice by their secretarial staff. The hospital services in the area can be relied upon to help the doctor in his task of caring for his patients. Relationships with community workers in the area are good. It would be surprising if these many favourable factors did not affect the workload of the partners in this practice. The extent to which the workload of this doctor differs from the average will be considered.

Doctor's Surgery Schedule

Monday	8.30–10.00; 11.30–12.30	16.30–18.00
Tuesday	Visits only	Half day
Wednesday	8.30–10.30; 11.00–12.00 (ante-natal)	17.00–18.00
Thursday	8.30–10.15	14.00–15.30
Friday	10.30–12.30	14.00–15.30; 16.30–18.00

Notes

1. Census of Population Reports (England and Wales) Office of Population Census and Surveys, London. General Register Office, Edinburgh. 1961 Census–social economic group tables published in April 1966. 1966 Census–economic activity tables. 1971 Census.
2. Whitfied, M.J. (1972) Relationship between year of registration and mobility. *Jnl. R.C.G.P.*, 22, 675-8.

5. DISEASE PREVALENCE AND HOSPITALS REFERRALS

The unusually low workload for the general practitioners in the Norton practice will be described in the next chapter. To put this in its proper perspective the question has to be asked whether there are any special factors making for a low incidence of disease or for a low incidence of consultation.

An unpolluted atmosphere, the absence of an influenza epidemic during the year or a high rate of referral to the local hospital are among the factors which would normally be expected to reduce the workload for the doctor. Were any such factors present in Norton at the time of the survey? Cleveland county is an area of high morbidity and mortality. There is considerable atmospheric pollution – it is one of the worst areas of the country in this respect. There is therefore no reason to suppose that the incidence of disease in the community served by the Norton medical centre is less than in Great Britain as a whole. It may well be greater.

There have been several studies of the clinical content of general practice according to the diagnosis made at each consultation.[1,2,3,4] Respiratory infections are commonest, usually followed by psychiatric illness. Marsh calculated an average frequency rating of all the groups which although not statistically precise gave an approximate overall picture of general practice.[5] He found that approximately 25 per cent of the consultations in general practice were for respiratory infections and one tenth for psychiatric illness.

In the present survey 25 per cent of the consultations were for respiratory infections and 14 per cent for psychiatric disease, thus suggesting that the practice was similar to the national average (Table 1). Upper respiratory tract infection was the commonest condition, accounting for 10 per cent of all consultations, and depression was second with 7 per cent of consultations (Table 2). Anxiety state was fifth. The system of recording which was used in the survey highlighted the true incidence of psychiatric illness because up to four diagnoses could be recorded at each consultation. At 35 per cent of consultations two or more diagnoses were discussed (Table 3). Doctors usually record the somatic illness present in the patient rather than its psychiatric sequelae if they are limited to the recording of one diagnosis per consultation.

An attempt was made to discover what proportion of patients in the practice required 'intensive care'. A record was made of patients who were seen twice or more in one day, three times in seven days or four times in twenty-eight days. One hundred and eighty-four patients,

6 per cent of the practice, received 'intensive care' during the year, and 69, just over 2 per cent were seen twice or more in one day for conditions ranging from profound heart failure to severe depression. The presence of an influenza epidemic can cause a very heavy workload in general practice. In December 1972 a particularly high workload was created by the influenza A England 42 virus in Cleveland, where 163 consultations were carried out for 'epidemic flu'.

Many of the simpler diagnostic routines are carried out by doctor or nurse in the practice side-room. Urinalysis, microscopy and various chemical tests on urine and faeces take place there. The extensive use of the hospital diagnostic facilities to which reference has been made in chapter 4 resulted in 1,193 patient referrals and these are shown in Table 4. Overall 43 per cent of this very large number of referrals carried out were found to be abnormal. Such tests would normally be expected to increase the workload of the general practitioner as once the investigations are completed the patient returns to his doctor for further advice and care.

The referral of patients to the out-patient and in-patient departments of the hospital for specialist opinion and care is one way in which a general practitioner can be relieved of responsibility for the diagnosis and treatment of disease. This was not the case in the Norton practice. The use made of the diagnostic facilities was one reason for this, as many tests are performed to check that there is no clinical disease. Once this is excluded it is not necessary to seek specialist opinion. The hospital referral rate was remarkably low; the proportion of patients referred to out-patient departments was only 38 per cent of the national average and that referred to the in-patient department was only 68 per cent (Tables 5 and 6). The low workload could not therefore be the result of a high referral rate – in fact, the low referral rate to the hospital would normally produce a heavy workload for the general practitioner.

Notes

1. Logan, W.P.D. and CUSHION, A.A. (1958) *General Register Office studies on medical and population subjects. No 14, Morbidity statistics from general practitioners.* HMSO, London.
2. Fry, J. (1966) *Profiles of Disease, A study in the Natural History of Common Diseases.* E. & S. Livingstone, London.
3. Dinwoodie, H.P. (1969) An elementary use of a computer for morbidity recording in general practice. *Health Bull.*, 1969, 27, 6-14.
4. Morrell, D.C. (1971) Expressions of morbidity in general practice. *Brit. Med. J.*, 1971, 2, 454-8.
5. Marsh, G.N. (1974) Team workload in general practice. MD thesis, University of Newcastle-upon-Tyne, 1974 (Not published).

6 FACTS AND FIGURES – THE WORKLOAD SURVEY IN THE NORTON PRACTICE

The workload created by the 3,137 patients on the doctor's list was very small. This was the most striking finding of the survey. The doctor had only 2.3 consultations per patient per year, which is one of the lowest reported consultation rates in the United Kingdom. He also made comparatively few visits, each patient receiving on average 0.4 visits during the year. The ratio of attendances to home visits was as high as five to one. The doctor saw 62 per cent of the patients on his list, these patients consulting on average 3.8 times. He visited 14 per cent of his patients and saw 58 per cent at the surgery (Tables 7-9).

Despite the low consultation rate, contact was made with a large proportion of households. All households with five or more members had some contact with the doctor and over 40 per cent were visited. Between 82 and 95 per cent of smaller families were contacted and well over 25 per cent visited during the year (Table 10).

Characteristics of Patients

A much heavier workload was created by women than by men. Not only did a larger proportion of female patients consult, but they consulted more frequently. The doctor saw 67 per cent of his female patients on average 4.1 times and 56 per cent of male patients 3.4 times. Women also received more home visits. The ratio of attendances to home visits was as low as four and a half to one for female patients compared with the high ratio of six to one for males. Twice as many of the doctor's visits were to women as to men (Tables 7-9).

The youngest age groups created the heaviest workload; 95 per cent of babies under one year old consulted on average five times, while 75 per cent of children aged between one and five years consulted three times. Patients over 65 years of age were the next highest consulting group with 70 per cent consulting on average four times during the year. Elderly patients created a heavier workload overall because there were many more patients in this age group (Table 11).

Although a large proportion of children under five received home visits, they did so less frequently than patients over forty-five years of age. Babies and patients over sixty-five received a greater proportion of home visits than patients in any other age group. The ratio of attendances to home visits was as low as one to one and a half for patients over sixty-five. Patients between forty-five and sixty-five years of age had the next lowest ratio, followed by the under fives. Older children and their parents had a much larger proportion of their consultations at the surgery. The survey demonstrated that the doctor's workload is heaviest for patients at the extremes of youth and age (Tables 12-14).

An examination of the proportion of patients who consulted the doctor during the year according to social class did not show statistically significant differences; a slightly lower proportion of patients in classes IV and V consulted than patients in the other classes. When attendances and visits were considered separately, the results were more significant. A much higher proportion of patients in social classes I and II attended the surgery during the year, while a slightly higher proportion of patients in classes IV and V were visited (Tables 15-17).

The most interesting results emerged when a study was made of those patients who consulted the doctor. Every member of the team made more contact with social class I and II households than with households of social classes IV and V (Table 18). Patients in classes IV and V consulted on average 4.3 times compared with an average rate of 3.5 for classes I and II. The lower-class patients also had a much lower ratio of attendances to visits, with an average of 3.9 consultations at the surgery to one home visit. By requiring more frequent consultations and a larger proportion of home visits, patients in classes IV and V created a heavy workload (Table 19).

Patients who had moved recently to the area were compared with those who had lived there for an appreciable time. A study was made of patients over eleven years of age who did not consult the doctor during the year and had registered since 1960. The figures suggest that the longer patients have been on the list, the less likely they are to consult the doctor. The group of patients who had registered recently contained a much higher proportion of consulters. They also had a low ratio of attendances to visits with four attendances to one home visit. Newly-arrived patients created a heavier workload than patients who had been in the area longer, a finding which adds statistical weight to the impression which many doctors have formed (Tables 20,21). These findings may result from the fact that migrants to an area will frequently only register with a doctor when they are ill and not when they arrive at their new address.

Doctor-Initiated Workload

The doctor recorded whether or not he had initiated the consultation with the patient. This was important as it has been found, notably in Aberdeen, that the general practitioner can control his own workload by regulating the number of follow-up consultations which he advises. There are inevitably some inaccuracies in the recording of doctor-initiated contacts but an endeavour was made to keep these to a minimum. Consultations were defined as 'doctor-initiated' only if the doctor gave a patient definite instructions to consult him on a specific day. If the doctor instructed the patient to consult him again only in certain circumstances, any such consultation was defined patient-initiated.

The doctor initiated more follow-up consultations with female than with male patients. This was probably due to the fact that ante-natal attendances are invariably initiated by the doctor. If patients between fifteen and forty-four years of age are excluded the doctor initiated more consultations with his male patients.

Babies under one year old and adults over forty-five years of age received many more follow-up consultations than patients in other age groups. Patients in social classes IV and V had a higher proportion of follow-up consultations than those in classes I and II (Tables 22-23).

Patients Causing the Heaviest Workload

The doctor's entire workload was created by 62 per cent of his patients. A very small proportion of the patients on his list caused a very large proportion of his work; half the total number of consultations were with 13 per cent of patients and a quarter with only 5 per cent.

The doctor visited 14 per cent of patients on his list but half his visits were to only 2 per cent. This is an important finding. A disproportionate amount of work is involved in a home visit compared with a surgery consultation. The fact that so few patients caused such a large proportion of visits means that a great deal of work was done for the benefit of a comparatively small number of people (Tables 24-26).

The doctor had no consultations with 38 per cent of his patients. A larger proportion of male than female patients did not consult. Very few babies under one year old and relatively few children under five years did not consult; the proportion of non-consulters between the ages of five to sixty-five varied little, and above that age it declined. A comparatively high proportion of babies and elderly people received home visits. There was no significant difference in the proportion of patients in each social class who were never visited, but a much greater proportion of class IV and V than class I and II patients never attended the surgery.

In contrast, a study was made of the 9 per cent of patients who received six or more consultations during the year. A larger proportion of female than male patients were in this category. Over 25 per cent of babies under one year consulted frequently. More patients in social classes IV and V than in I and II were frequent consulters (Tables 27, 28).

In all practices some patients are well known to the doctor for the frequency with which they consult. This practice is no exception. It was therefore decided to examine the characteristics of the twenty male and twenty female patients who received the highest number of consultations during 1972.

The twenty male patients consulted on average sixteen times. The great majority were in the second half of life. Six were in social classes I and II. Depression, asthma, alcoholism and social problems were more common among this group than in the practice as a whole.

The average consultation rate for the twenty female patients was eighteen. Only one patient, a baby, was not in the second half of life. One was in classes I and II. Twelve of these women had severe psychiatric illnesses, while acute and chronic illnesses were also present. Pregnant women were not included in the detailed study but if they had been then thirteen of the most frequent consulters were expecting a child. Their inclusion would have raised the average consultation rate from eighteen to over twenty-two.

The chronic housebound sick create a very heavy workload for the general practitioner. They consisted of the thirty patients who were permanently on the doctor's visiting list and were likely to remain there in the foreseeable future. Most of these patients had been on the visiting list for several years. The workload created by the twenty-two female patients was three times as great as that created by the males, which was probably due to the greater longevity of females. There were chronic housebound sick patients in every social class. Twenty-six of these thirty patients were over sixty-five years of age. Congestive heart failure, osteo-arthritis, advanced rheumatoid arthritis and crippling respiratory disease were the conditions which made it impossible for these patients to lead active lives and necessitated home visits. Several suffered from two of these diseases.

The Season of the Year and the Day of the Week

The total consultative workload remained remarkably constant throughout the year; only in the summer did the proportion of consultations fall and then only to 23 per cent of the total for the year. Attendances were similarly unaffected by seasonal change, except that there were slightly more surgery attendances in spring than in winter. Winter was by far the busiest season for home visiting; as many as 38 per cent of requests for home visits were made during that quarter. This meant that more effort was required of the doctor during the winter months. The doctor initiated fewer attendances during the summer than at other times, presumably because of his own absences on holiday (Table 29).

Over half the total number of consultations took place on Mondays and Wednesdays and 33 per cent on Thursdays and Fridays. Only 6 per cent of consultations took place on Tuesday, the doctor's half-day. Eight patients consulted on average each Tuesday. The workload was also very light at weekends with only four consultations on Saturdays and between one and two on Sundays.

Wednesday was the busiest day in terms of the number of patients who were seen, but Monday was the heaviest visiting day (Table 30). Patients initiated more work on a Monday than on any other day of the week, but even then an average of only two visits was requested. The average number of consultations for the five week days was twenty-seven.

The Saturday morning surgery was used more frequently by men than by women. Men also received more visits at the weekend. Children, in addition to their high total attendances, had a disproportionately high number of attendances on Saturdays and Sundays. Patients in social classes I and II were more inclined to use the Saturday morning surgery than those in classes IV and V.

The Nurse's Workload

The strong team which supported the doctor in his work has already been described. What proportion of work did these staff undertake?

After nearly 4 per cent of his surgery consultations and after just over 13 per cent of visits the doctor delegated the immediate subsequent care of the patient to nurse. In this way, he referred 4 per cent of the patients who attended the surgery and 27 per cent of those he visited. The care of adults was delegated to a nurse more frequently than that of children, and social class I and II patients were referred to her more frequently than patients in other social groups.

Nurses undertook 1,924 consultations during the year, which is about 25 per cent of the number undertaken by the doctor. They had a heavy visiting workload with twice as many home visits as consultations at the surgery. All their work was for 17 per cent of the patients on the list and a half for only 1 per cent. Nevertheless they did contact a large number of households. Nurses saw patients from 30 per cent of households with two or more members and as many as 57 per cent of households with five members (Table 10).

Follow-up work for patients seen initially by the doctor formed a large proportion of the nurses' work. The follow-up of chronically ill patients caused half their workload while the follow-up of acutely ill patients caused a fifth (Table 31). Senility as defined by the nurse was the most common condition requiring follow-up care. Patients suffering from anaemias also caused a sizeable proportion of this work because of the diagnostic venepunctures and therapeutic routines necessitated by anaemic conditions (Table 32).

The acute conditions seen by the nurse in the first instance were mainly respiratory infections such as influenza, bronchitis and tonsillitis. Minor injuries were often attended by the nurse. During the year the clinical treatment and diagnostic techniques which she undertook included 435 injections, 342 dressings, 251 venepunctures and 114 blood pressure checks.

The Health Visitor's Workload

The health visitor carried out about a third of the number of consultations which were undertaken by the nurse. She had a very high ratio of attendances to home visits, with nearly seven attendances to one visit. All her work was caused by 6 per cent of the patients on the list and a half by 1 per cent. She did however have contact with a larger proportion of households; for example, she had consultations with members from a quarter of four-person households (Table 10). She saw a higher proportion of patients from classes I and II than from other social classes (Table 18). Over half of her consultations were with mothers seeking advice about the general care of their babies. This was because patients were familiar with her traditional role in child welfare clinics and because nurses did a large proportion of the visiting of elderly people.

The small number of consultations carried out by the health visitor does not reflect a limited need for her services. Unfortunately there is a shortage of health visitors in Cleveland county, which means that one health visitor must meet the needs of 15,000 patients. She had only 2.5 hours per week available for every thousand patients in the practice. Nurses were available for 11.4 hours per 1,000 patients per week. The consultation rate for the entire doctor, nurse and health visitor team was 3.1 consultations per patient per year (Table 33).

The Midwife's Workload

The number of formal referrals to the midwife was too small to yield useful findings. She occasionally undertook the follow-up of illnesses in pregnant patients who were not in hospital and chased up patients who were not consulting regularly at the ante-natal clinic. She took a prominent part in the ante-natal care of patients, deputising completely for the doctor when he was on holiday or study leave. Both midwife and doctor normally attended ante-natal clinics and shared the task of examining patients.

The midwife attended patients during labour and delivered them in the 'very early discharge unit' of the local hospital. She called the doctor for attendance during delivery and at other times if problems arose. She then looked after these patients at home during the puerperal period. She also looked after patients who were discharged after forty-eight hours from the district maternity hospital. The doctor visited these patients regularly.

The Social Worker

Patients were referred to the social worker on twenty-five occasions. Occasionally health visitor and social worker cooperated in the assessment and care of patients with social problems. Included in this work was the overall assessment of a problem family containing a near-alcoholic mother, an unemployable asthmatic son and a brother with symptoms of schizophrenia; arrangements for the provision of a lift to the bedroom and other mechanical aids for a young mother who was rapidly becoming crippled by multiple sclerosis and the assessment of a request for termination of pregnancy for social reasons.

7 LOW WORKLOAD – SATISFIED PATIENTS?

The very low workload created for the doctor by his 3,137 patients raises some important questions. The doctor had on average only 2.3 consultations with each patient during the year. His visiting workload was particularly small with a ratio of surgery attendances to home visits as high as five to one, the average for the north-east of England being three to one. This low visiting workload was mainly due to the supplementation of visiting by the nurse who had twice as many consultations at patients' homes as at the surgery. But are patients who see their doctor so seldom and may well receive visits from the nurse in his place satisfied with this kind of medical and nursing care?

It must be emphasised that despite the very low consultation rate for each patient and the fact that a very small percentage of patients created a large amount of the doctor's work, a very high proportion of *households* were contacted. This consideration of the contact made with households rather than patients is very relevant in assessing how far the doctor was in touch with his patients and it is probable that some of the satisfaction which a patient feels with the doctor's care may well reflect his satisfaction with the care seen to be given to other members of his household.

Various factors have been shown to be associated with a low workload for the doctor. An area of low morbidity, a high proportion of males or a low proportion of children and old people on the practice list, an unusual distribution of social class, or a very stable population are all relevant in this respect. None of these factors was operative in the practice in Norton. Another reason for a low workload can be a high rate of referral to hospital, which again was not the case. Even a fairly severe influenza epidemic did not cause the workload to be high, indicating that in years without an epidemic it would have been even lower.

It is probably safe to assume that the quality of care which a doctor gives his patients affects his workload. If it were cursory, superficial, dismissive and of a low clinical standard then the workload might well be small. It would be pleasant to be able to demonstrate that this was not the case in the Norton practice, but despite much discussion[1,2] and some tentative suggestions[3] no defined and acceptable standards of the quality of clinical care in general practice have been specified. Until this is done, no evaluation can be made in this or any other practice. Some doctors believe that practices with a low workload could be achieving this by adopting somewhat intransigent attitudes to such psychiatric problems as anxiety state, depression and neurosis.

The fact that 14 per cent of consultations in this practice included a discussion of a psychiatric problem is some evidence that this attitude was not adopted by the general practitioner.

There are other indications that the standard of care was satisfactory. Just under 6 per cent of all patients received 'intensive care' during the year (see page 65 of MS) and the nature of the care given to patients who saw the doctor frequently also suggests reasonable standards.[4] The referral rate to diagnostic departments was high with a large proportion of abnormal findings yet there was a low rate of referral to consultants. This suggests that while clinical care was undertaken thoroughly, responsibility for managing illness remained with the general practitioner.

There are two factors operating in the practice which are known to be associated with a low consultation rate. First, the list size is considerably greater than average with 700 patients more than on the average list. This no doubt contributes to some extent to the low consultation rate, although this must be distinguished from the overall workload of the doctor. Second, the practice runs a very sophisticated appointment system, aiming to provide 'same day' access to the patient's own doctor on most days. How well this works and how satisfied patients are with the system are relevant questions which have to be considered.

The proportion of work which a doctor himself initiates has been shown to have some effect on his overall workload. Other studies have attempted to assess this.[5,6,7] The proportion in Norton was comparatively low at 39 per cent.

If the general practitioner is established, experienced and clinically confident, he should be able to assess which patients require follow-up treatment. This should only be necessary either when the patient is unable to determine whether he is better or not, or for the monitoring of severe or chronic illness. Many patients are quite happy to get better without further consultations provided they receive a thorough assessment from the doctor they know and trust at the initial consultation and have been given a short summary of the course and duration of the illness. This careful initial explanation should also enable the patient to know whether he needs further consultation after a specified time. Such clinical advice is an aspect of health education. It is necessary to ask whether it satisfies the patient as effectively as it reduces the workload for the doctor.

The doctor must know 'his' patients and the patients 'their' doctor if the system of educating the patient to follow up the course of his illness is to work well. Much effort is saved for the doctor if he is caring for familiar patients often with familiar problems whose background is well known to him. Lengthy diagnostic and consultative rituals are only necessary for unfamiliar faces. It is thought that in this practice the care of individual patients by individual doctors has helped to curtail the workload in a way which would not have been possible if patients remained free to move from one doctor to another.

The concept of the single-handed practice is adhered to under the umbrella of the group. When patients were first asked to consult their own doctor whenever possible, some readjustment had to be made to the surgery appointment system to facilitate this. The upheaval has been found to be well worth while in terms of the resultant saving of effort. Telephone consultations, repeat prescriptions for continuing illnesses, the process of accustoming patients to a particular way of working, especially in relation to home visits, and the role of other members of the health care team are some of the adjustments which have been made easier by increasing personalised care. It must be asked whether this system of care is as acceptable to the patient as it is to the doctor.

The amount of work which was delegated to the team is the main measurable finding in the survey. In order to achieve integration, the team meets informally for about fifteen minutes each morning. During that short time work is allocated, cases are discussed and treatment is agreed. Contact can continue during the day, particularly between nurse and doctor, as and when problems arise. Thus duplication of work is avoided and each member of the team can operate at a level appropriate to his or her skills.

State registered nurses are supported by the state enrolled nurse and the bath attendant. This relieves them of many of the tasks which they have undertaken in the past and gives them time to carry out some of the care of patients which was previously undertaken by the doctor. Nurses are always on duty at the surgery to see patients who have not taken their problems to the doctor. New requests for the doctor to call at the house are undertaken by the attached local authority nurses if, after a careful assessment of both the patients' records and the information received by trained receptionists, this seems appropriate. The nurse is provided with what would appear to be the appropriate signed prescription which she can leave with the patient if she is able to confirm that it is indicated. Any alternative prescription can be suggested to the doctor by the nurse after seeing the patient but in that case a messenger will need to get such a prescription from the surgery. It is very possible in that eventuality that the doctor himself will also feel obliged to visit the patient. At the time of the survey only about 5 per cent of the nurses' consultations were new visits of this type. A fifth of the nurses' workload involved the follow-up and management of acute illness, most of this in the homes of patients who had previously been seen by the doctor and whom the doctor would have needed to see again if it were not for her support. The doctor was also able to delegate almost all diagnostic routines such as venepunctures, ECGs and swabs after consultations in the surgery or at the patient's home. However, the largest part of the nurse's workload was the follow-up of chronic illness. The many ways in which nurses have undertaken or shared the care of patients has made an enormous contribution to the lessening of the doctor's workload. It is essential to discover whether patients mind having nurses to share care with the doctor, monitor their progress, and undertake various techniques and procedures. Above all it must be asked whether they resent being visited by the nurse when they had asked for the doctor to call.

If patients are well satisfied and are accustomed to accept the ministrations of the nurse, more of the consultative work could be undertaken by her. In order to facilitate this the surgery card which patients receive upon registering now contains information about the availability of nurses for minor problems or for those problems which patients themselves consider could be dealt with appropriately by the nurse. (This process was hindered by the lack of privacy in the nurses' treatment room which was also too large to encourage the establishment of consultative rapport. Recent building developments have rectified this.) The doctor is prepared to sign prescriptions ordered by nurses he knows and trusts for conditions whose diagnosis and management he knows are within their capabilities. It is pertinent to recall that doctors in most practices sign prescriptions for patients who recount symptoms to receptionists ('sticky eye', 'tonsillitis again' etc.).

It is very important that nurses who undertake this new kind of care either at the surgery or in the patient's home should be able to attend courses carefully designed to help them adapt and train for this task. Such training is not yet generally available and the steps being taken by the Joint Board of Clinical Nursing Studies to establish courses are welcome. A group designing a syllabus for nurses working in primary health care teams might find the analysis of acute conditions and chronic illness which nurses deal with in the Norton practice useful (Table 32).

There were very few direct referrals to the health visitor as she was already involved with the care of babies and children in the practice through the well-baby clinic and the pursuit of her statutory duties. Many of her appointments were initiated by patients who were well aware of her role and already knew her. Over half of her work was general health advice involving the care of babies at the well-baby clinic. She also carried out most of the developmental pediatric programme. Much of the health work with problem families and the aged for which health visitors have been responsible in the past is now undertaken by the social worker and the district nursing team. It is however apparent that her activities could further minimise the doctor's workload if her role were expanded to include the care of certain clinical problems such as obesity, enuresis and behaviour disturbances. Certainly nurses of this standard and training should be given scope to extend more effective health counselling to groups of patients who are at risk. An assessment of patients' satisfaction with the work she already undertakes is necessary before this development takes place.

The effect of social class on the workload of both the nurse and health visitor was assessed in the survey. Social class has become a subject of discussion in relation to team care. There has always been some anxiety that members of the team other than the doctor would be used to a greater extent by patients in social classes IV and V than by those in classes I and II who, it has been assumed, would insist on having direct contact with the doctor. It has also been thought that it might be easier for the doctor to delegate the care of social class IV and V patients to other members of the health care team. In this survey the very converse was found to be the case. In both sexes a higher proportion of class I and II patients have consultations with the nurse than of any other social class. The figures for visiting are not conclusive but give no indication that visits by the nurse are unacceptable to class I and II patients. It may be that a higher proportion of patients in these classes have a better understanding of the way to use the services of all members of the health care team. An examination of social class differences is certainly important in any consideration of the satisfaction which patients feel with the care given to them by the nurse and health visitor.

When the role of the midwife was considered in the survey, it became apparent that doctor and midwife were duplicating care in the antenatal and puerperal periods. Practices which have fully developed 'shared care' systems must be lessening the doctor's workload. Such practices find that the midwife who is seen to be closely linked with the doctor can deal expertly with the minor discomforts and problems of pregnancy and can give much of the necessary reassurance to anxious patients about problems which may seem very worrying but are in fact normal and easily dealt with.

The complete physical examination and assessment of the patients at the beginning of the pregnancy must be carried out by the doctor himself. After this there is no doubt that most of the routine care of patients who are not at risk could be undertaken solely by the midwife who could refer problems to the doctor when they arise. The doctor would play a larger part in the care of patients, particularly those at risk, towards the end of pregnancy. During the puerperium the routine care of the patient could also be undertaken by the midwife, the doctor confining his attention to high-risk patients. He would also visit each patient on the fifth to seventh day after the birth to carry out a complete physical examination of the baby, this being of paramount importance. The midwife could also visit patients who asked to see the doctor in their homes during pregnancy or the puerperal period provided she could communicate with the doctor without delay if it should be necessary.

Care during the confinement is probably shared to a reasonable extent in the practice and there is little need for change, although it is feasible that the midwife could be instructed in the repair of minor lacerations of the perineum in addition to carrying out episiotomies. In good obstetric care the presence of two trained personnel, in this case the doctor and the midwife, is desirable to maintain the high quality of response to obstetric emergency which modern general practice demands.

If shared care is to be extended in this field it is essential that doctor, midwife and patient should all understand the new system. All too often the patient is not sufficiently initiated into such changes and loses confidence. The midwife must be seen to be the trained, reliable worker which she in fact is. It is also important to discover how far patients would favour an expansion of her role.

The patient satisfaction survey, which is described in the second part of this book, answers this and the many other questions which have been raised. An attempt has been made here to describe a modern Primary Health Care Team, detailing its operational and clinical work in a practice which is a fairly typical cross-section of the English population in an urban area. How satisfied patients are with this kind of care with its resultant low workload for the doctor and extensive use of nursing staff will be discussed. But what of the doctor himself?

Integrated team work of the kind described is the pattern for the future. The increasing development of health centres and large group practices will speed up this change. It has been shown that this type of care can result in a low workload for the doctor and a low rate of referral to hospital.

The average list size of 2,400 patients may well become too small to occupy the time of the established general practitioner but the particular characteristics of the population served by individual practices should, in future, be given increasing consideration. In addition some doctors will want to spend time teaching new entrants to general practice as members of the various trainee schemes which are now established, and others will wish to pursue clinical or operational research. Some may wish to undertake more work in hospitals or increase their commitments in preventive care and health education. But there is also the distinct possibility that in future general practitioners will consider it reasonable to have longer lists than are acceptable at present and indeed need these in order to satisfy their clinical interests. The manpower requirements of general practice in a team setting will be different from those in the past for all members of the team but for the doctors themselves it seems that the requirements will be lower than is generally thought at present. The implications of this change involve major issues of public policy which are well beyond the scope of this study.

Notes

1. Buck, C. *et al* (1974) A framework for good primary medical care – the measurement and achievement of quality. *Jnl. R.C.G.P.*, 1974, 24, 599.

2. Marson, W.S. *et al* (1973) Measuring the quality of general practice, *Jnl. R.C.G.P.*, 1973, 23, 23.
3. Hodgkin, G.K. (1973) Evaluating the doctor's work. *Jnl. R.C.G.P.*, 1973, 23, 759.
4. Marsh, G.N. (1974) Team workload in general practice. M.D. thesis, University of Newcastle-upon-Tyne, 1974 (not published).
5. Morrell, D.C. *et al* (1970) Patterns of demand in general practice, *Jnl. R.C.G.P.*, 1970, 19, 331-42.
6. Royal College of General Practitioners (1970) *A study of general practitioners' workload in South Wales*, 1965-66. Reports from General Practice No.XII, 1970.
7. Richardson, I.M. *et al* (1973) A study of general practitioners' consultations in north-east Scotland. *Jnl. R.C.G.P.*,1973, 23, 132-42.

APPENDIX MECHANICS OF DATA COLLECTION FOR THE WORKLOAD SURVEY

The Newcastle-upon-Tyne Regional Hospital Board funded the survey by a grant which enabled the practice to employ a full-time research secretary. The statistical officer of the board, Mr. Angus McNay, acted as statistical consultant to the study and the data was analysed on the board's ICL 1902A computer. During the three months preceding the study, the forms for collecting information were designed and evaluated in a pilot survey.

It was decided to provide a record on computer cards of every item of medical care provided by the doctor, the health visitor and the nurses so that all aspects of care would be available for analysis. The computer was to store all operational and clinical data concerning the 3,100 patients receiving their medical care from one doctor and his team. The reception and secretarial staff were briefed to ensure that records were made of any items of care rendered to these patients by other doctors in the practice.

All patients on the doctor's list at the beginning of 1972 or registering in that year were included in the survey. This meant that the number of patients on the list was slightly larger than the number who were in the doctor's care at any one time. Some patients left the practice during the year while others joined later, so that neither of these groups was on the list for the whole of 1972. A nominal list for 1 July 1972 contained 2,951 names compared with the 3,137 on the survey list. The procedure adopted was considered preferable to any other as it ensured that all work done for patients during the year was included in the survey. There was no difference in the age, social class or sex structure of the patients on the nominal list and those in the study. The statistical consultant did not consider that the differences between the two lists would affect any of the aspects of workload which were being evaluated.

Morrell (1970)[1] has described the difficulty in determining list size accurately. It is known that nationally there is an inflation of practice lists when compared to the number of patients for which practices are actually responsible. This occurs because patients who move to new areas sometimes fail to register with new practices and therefore their names are not removed from the list of the practice which previously cared for them. It also occasionally happens that names are not removed from a practice list because of clerical errors by the executive councils. Provision is made for the removal of the names of patients who die or emigrate from the doctor's list but here too the machinery does not always work properly.

In order to reduce the number of these 'ghost' patients for the purpose of this study, a careful scrutiny was made of all patients' records entered in the survey. Several patients were excluded when checks with the executive council showed that they had left the area. A further check was made at the end of the year when the survey had been completed. This took the form of reviewing the records of the 900 patients with whom no contact had been made. This led to the conclusion that presumably a tenth of these patients were no longer in the area or were no longer convered by the practice. It thus appears that the list may have been inflated by some 3 per cent, rather less than the 5 per cent by which the average practice list is inflated. Computers have been used in few practices in Britain for storing information about patients.[1,2,3,4,5,6] It is therefore thought to be of interest to outline the mechanics of transfer of the information received from general practice records on to the computer.

It was essential that the system of recording should involve the doctor and the other members of the team in the minimum of extra effort. All the records were kept by the research secretary, the doctor merely having to note the date and place of consultation on the standard surgery record card and state in his clinical notes the diagnosis or diagnoses considered at each consultation. A ring was put round each new diagnosis. The record cards were issued to the doctor for all home visits as well as for surgery attendances. This was in any case the normal practice for the group but additional care had to be taken to make certain that the cards were intelligible to the research secretary.

Extra code numbers in front of the date indicated whether the consultation had been initiated by the doctor or the patient. A code letter showed whether the consultation was followed by referral to a nurse (N) or a health visitor (HV). The research secretary could thus extract all information required for computer storage and analysis by scanning the standard record cards (page 73). The receptionist and filing staff had been carefully instructed before the commencement of the survey to ensure that patients' record cards reached the research secretary after each consultation.

The standard record envelope has on the front the patient's name, address, sex, and date of birth and where this was missing it was obtained from the executive council (page 74). All these data were recorded on initial form I which also had space for recording change of name, change of address and the date of leaving the list if this occurred during the survey (page 75).

The occupations of 70 per cent of heads of households were obtained by enquiring from an adult member of the household. These questions were asked at the time of a consultation in the six months preceding the survey and up to March 1972. The other 30 per cent of heads of households received a letter from the doctor asking them for this information. To this two thirds replied giving their occupations. The remaining 10 per cent were classified from the doctor's knowledge of his patients, from the streets in which they lived and the type of house which they occupied. The heads of households according to their occupations were grouped into five social classes following the Registrar General's social class list. Social class I is the highest, containing barristers, architects and other 'professional' classes while V is the lowest, reserved for unskilled labourers. The social class of the head was attributed to all members of the household.

At a later stage it was decided that the number of patients in social classes I, II, IV and V were probably too small to make statistically valid comparisons. For this reason, social classes I and II, and classes IV and V, were combined, thereby reducing the number of social classes to three. This incidentally minimised the effect of errors in the classification. The most interesting as well as the most obvious findings were in any case expected to be in differences between social classes I and II as a group and classes IV and V as a group.

It would have been desirable to show the patient's marital status on initial form I but after careful consideration this classification was omitted. The marital status of patients frequently changes without this coming to the doctor's attention, so that any record would rapidly become faulty. In any case, as this characteristic is not shown on the record card, it would have been a major task to ascertain the marital status of all patients above the age of sixteen. It was also not anticipated that a study would be undertaken of the effects of marital status of either the utilisation of medical care or the doctor's workload.

The initial form I also incorporated a code indicating that a patient was chronically housebound and receiving routine visits from the doctor. This particular group of patients whose names were extracted from the doctor's visiting book was singled out for special study.

Initial form I was completed for all patients on the list on 31 December 1971 and for those patients who joined the list during 1972 at the time of their registration. An additional form was made out for all patients leaving the list in the course of 1972.

A street index of the practice was made out which made it possible to place patients into household groups each of which was given a number. The patient's household number the ward code (from the local authority map) and the distance of the household from the surgery – as the crow flies – were recorded on a household coding sheet. The pilot surveys had shown that it would have been difficult and unreliable to codify types of accommodation. Coding of the distance of the household's residence from a bus stop and the number of buses needed to take the patient to the surgery were similarly abandoned. Under present economic conditions, the use of a car is for many patients probably a more important factor than the bus routes in considering the ease with which the patient can get to the surgery; the value of information relating to bus routes was therefore considered of secondary importance.

The research secretary received from a receptionist after each consultation the standard NHS record envelope. She recorded the particulars of the contact on a specially designed surgery attendance card or home visit card (page 77). The number of the patient, the household number and the social class of the patients were shown on the envelope. Where the contact took place, by whom it was initiated, the date, the code number of the diagnosis and whether consultation was with the patient's own doctor were all entered on the appropriate cards.

The research secretary coded the diagnosis according to the Royal College of General Practitioners' classification of morbidity. This is a shortened version of the international classification of diseases and causes of death based on the frequency of these diseases in general practice in Britain. A supplementary list of diagnoses not identified in the RCGP's classification was drawn up specifically for the survey to record more detailed diagnoses and to reduce such classifications as 'other diseases of . . . . ' It was possible to make a diagnosis at each consultation as the RCGP's classification allows for a 'symptom' as well as an 'illness' diagnosis. A decision at the consultation to refer the patient to a nurse, health visitor, midwife, social worker or industrial medical officer was also entered on the card.

If the patient was referred to hospital as an in-patient or an out-patient a carbon copy of the referral letter was used to make an entry on a hospital contact sheet. The urgency of the referral and the main diagnosis were also noted. Hospital discharge letters coming to the practice were analysed and all in-patient treatment was also recorded. The laboratory and radiology reports from hospitals, any diagnosed abnormality and all diagnostic referrals were similarly recorded on the hospital contact sheet (page 78).

The health visitor and the local authority nurses recorded as routine for the local authority health department only the number of patients they had seen. For the purpose of the survey they had to record additional information. The nurses employed by the partners normally kept no formal records of any kind. All the five nursing members of the team, as part of the survey, recorded the place at which their work was carried out and the nature of the work they undertook on special sheets which provided a complete account of the services they rendered to the patients (page 79).

In-patients obstetric care in the general practitioner unit was noted on a special sheet so that an analysis of the work could be carried out.

For the purpose of giving a complete picture of the doctor's workload, including his work for other partners, a 'casual sheet' was completed for each patient seen from another doctor's list. This showed whether the consultation was at home or at the surgery and whether the patient was a temporary resident or normally on the list of another doctor in the practice.

The research secretary spent approximately three quarters of the working week entering information on the various forms which, after completion, were sent to the statistical department of the Newcastle-upon-Tyne Regional Hospital Board. There, they were checked for consistency and corrected if required. Thereafter, the data were transferred on to punch cards and analysed by the computer. After the survey had been in operation for six months, preliminary print-outs were run off. These made it possible to evaluate the results of the survey. As a result of this evaluation errors and omissions in the organisation of the survey and the recording of the data were corrected whenever this proved possible.

Notes

1. Morrell, D.C. *et al* (1971) Symptoms in general practice. *Jnl. R.C.G.P.*, 21,32.
2. Ockenden, J.M. and Bodenham, K.E. (1970) *Focus on Medical Computer Development.* Oxford University Press, London.
3. Dinwoodie, H.P. (1970) Simple computer facilities in general practice – a study of the problems involved. *Jnl. R.C.G.P.* 19, 269.
4. Gruer, K.T. (1972) Livingston New Town – using a computer for general practice records. *Jnl. R.C.G.P.*, 22,100.
5. Johnson, R.A. (1971) *World Medicine,* 6, 72.
6. Abrams, M.E. (1972) Health Services and the Computer. Real time computing in general practice. *Health Trends*, 1972, 4, 1, 18.

Patients Record Card

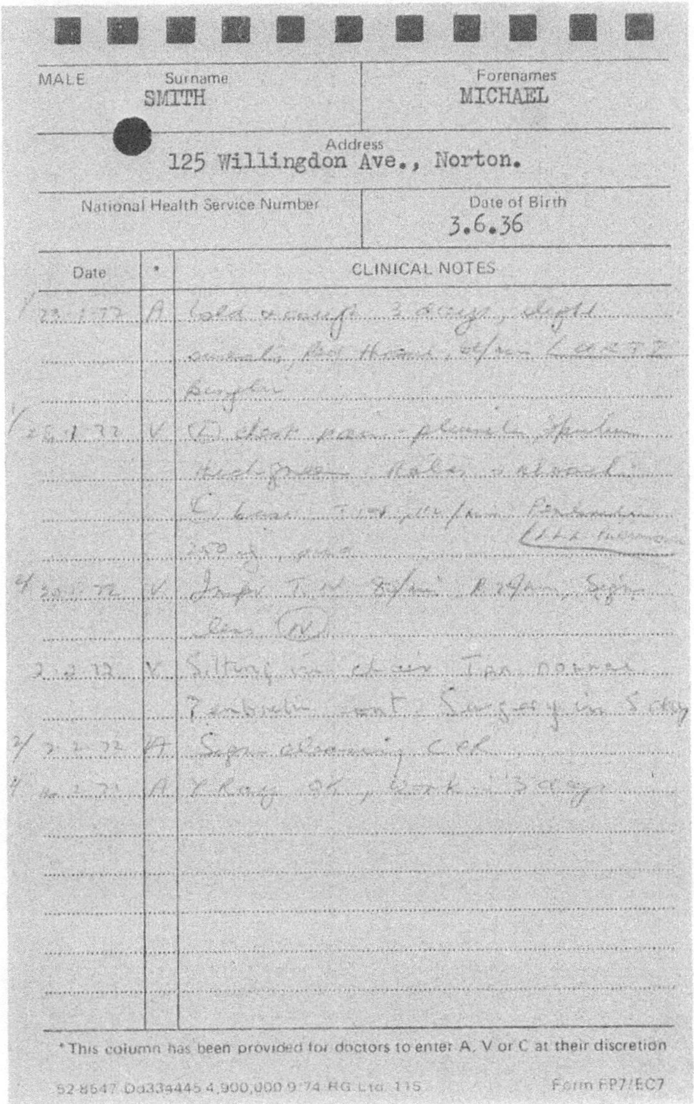

MALE

Surname: SMITH

Forenames: MICHAEL

Address: 125 Willingdon Ave., Norton.

National Health Service Number:

Date of Birth: 3.6.36

Date	*	CLINICAL NOTES
[illegible]	A	[illegible]
[illegible]	V	[illegible]
[illegible]	V	[illegible]
[illegible]	V	[illegible]
[illegible]	A	[illegible]
[illegible]	A	[illegible]

*This column has been provided for doctors to enter A, V or C at their discretion

52-8647 Dd334445 4,900,000 9/74 RG Ltd. 115 Form FP7/EC7

Record Envelope and enclosed Record Card

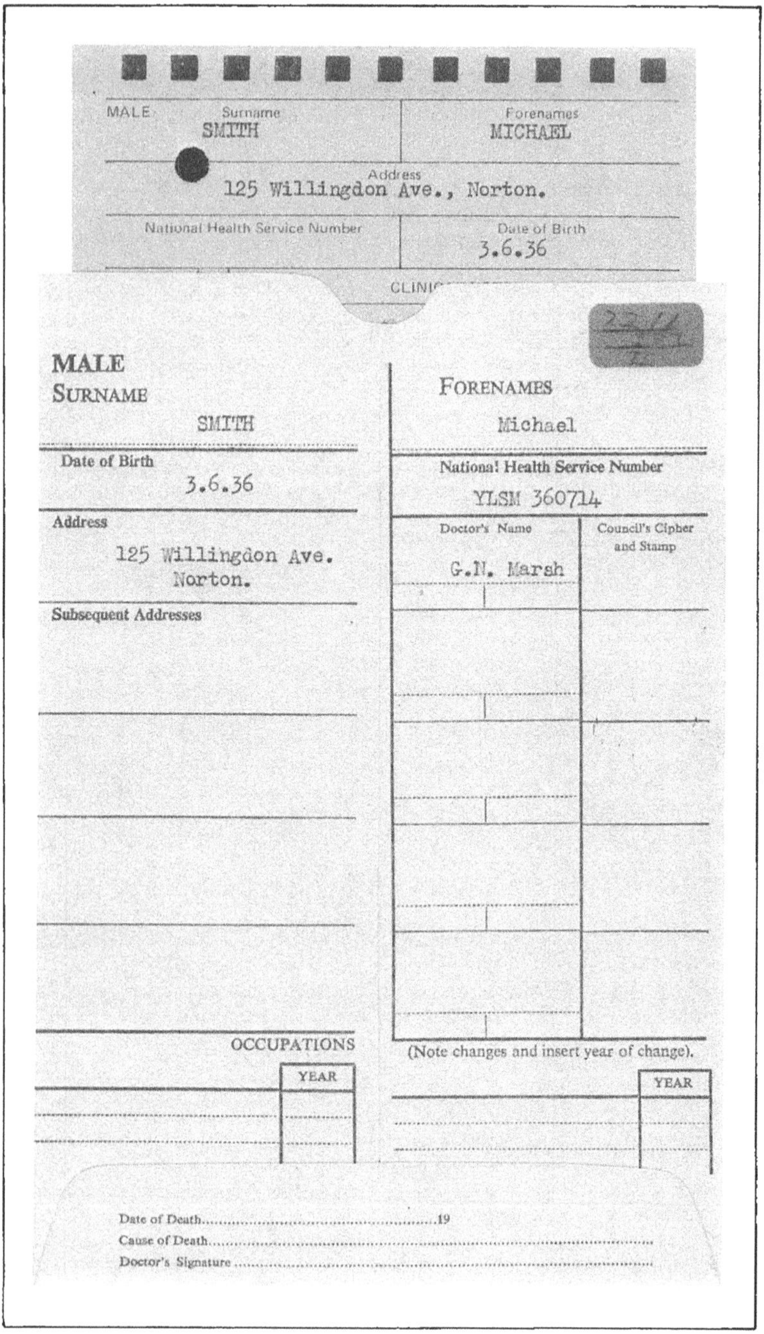

MALE
Surname SMITH
Forenames MICHAEL
Address 125 Willingdon Ave., Norton.
National Health Service Number
Date of Birth 3.6.36

MALE
SURNAME
SMITH

FORENAMES
Michael

Date of Birth
3.6.36

National Health Service Number
YLSM 360714

Address
125 Willingdon Ave.
Norton.

Doctor's Name
G.N. Marsh

Council's Cipher and Stamp

Subsequent Addresses

OCCUPATIONS

YEAR

(Note changes and insert year of change).

YEAR

Date of Death 19
Cause of Death ....
Doctor's Signature ....

GENERAL PRACTICE WORK LOAD STUDY Initial Form 1

PATIENT'S CHRISTIAN NAME: ..Michael.....................................

SURNAME (1) .....SMITH.....................................

SURNAME (2) ....

PATIENT'S ADDRESS (1) 125 Willingdon Avenue, NORTON...............

....

ADDRESS (2) ....

....

ADDRESS (3) ....

....

Form Type		1	1
Patient Number		2-5	2 2 1 1
Sex	Male = 1 Female = 2	6	1
Date of Birth		7-12	0 3 0 6 3 6
Date Joined List		13-18	1 1 0 3 2 9
On Chronic Visit List	Yes = 1 No = 2	19	2
Social Class		20	2
ADDRESS:			
(1) At beginning of survey:	Household code	21-23	5 3 7
(2) 1st change	Date	24-29	
	Household code	30-32	
(3) 2nd change	Date	33-38	
	Household code	39-41	
Date off list if appropriate		42-47	
Date Form Completed		48-53	0 2 0 1 7 2

General Practice Workload Study *Surgery Attendance Cards*

Form Type	To be punched on each card produced	1	3
Patient Number		2-5	2 2 1 1

column numbers	6-29	6-29	6-29	6-29
Date	2 3 0 1			
Initiated	1			
Nurse				
Midwife				
H.V.				
Social Worker/H.W.O.				
I.M.O.				
1st Diagnosis	2 4 0			
2nd Diagnosis				
3rd Diagnosis				
4th Diagnosis				
Code 1 if diagnosis pending				
Code 1 if GNM, otherwise 0	1			

Column numbers	6-29	6-29	6-29	6-29
Date				
Initiated				
Nurse				
Midwife				
H.V.				
Social Worker/H.W.O.				
I.M.O.				
1st Diagnosis				
2nd Diagnosis				
3rd Diagnosis				
4th Diagnosis				
Code 1 if diagnosis pending				
Code 1 if GNM, otherwise 0				

General Practice Workload Study *Home Visit Card*

Form Type	To be punched on each card produced	1	4
Patient Number		2-5	2 2 1 1

Column numbers	6 - 29	6 - 29	6 - 29	6 - 29
Date	2 8 0 1	3 0 0 1		
Initiated	1	2		
Nurse		✓		
Midwife				
H.V.				
Social Worker/M.W.O.				
I.M.O.				
1st Diagnosis	2 4 6	2 4 6		
2nd Diagnosis				
3rd Diagnosis				
4th Diagnosis				
Code 1 if diagnosis pending				
Code 1 if GNM, otherwise 0	1	1		

Column numbers	6 - 29	6 - 29	6 - 29	6 - 29
Date				
Initiated				
Nurse				
Midwife				
H.V.				
Social Worker/M.W.O.				
I.M.O.				
1st Diagnosis				
2nd Diagnosis				
3rd Diagnosis				
4th Diagnosis				
Code 1 if diagnosis pending				
Code 1 if GNM, otherwise 0				

Form Type	To be punched on each card produced	1	5
Patient Number		2-5	2 2 1 1

Col. Nos.	6 - 32	6 - 32	6 - 32	6 - 32
In-patient				
Date of Admission				
Source				
Diagnosis				
Discharge Date				
Out-patient				
Date of Referral				
Source				
Diagnosis				
Diagnostic				
Date	0 7 0 2			
Type and Normality N = Normal A = Abnormal	X C N			

Col. Nos.	6 - 32	6 - 32	6 - 32	6 - 32
In-patient				
Date of Admission				
Source				
Diagnosis				
Discharge Date				
Out-patient				
Date of Referral				
Source				
Diagnosis				
Diagnostic				
Date				
Type and Normality N = Normal A = Abnormal				

Health Visitors' Form

NAME	M Form
	Nurse
	DATE
Home/Surgery	(insert H or S)
New Acute	
F.U. Acute	
F.U. Chronic	
Post. Hospital	
Other	
G.N. Care	
Advice	
Dressings	
B.P. Check	
Cervical Smear	
E.C.G.	
Vitalometer	
Venepuncture	
Immunology	
Therapeutic Inject.	
Desens. Inject.	
Ear Syringe	
Other	
DIAGNOSIS	
OFFICE USE ONLY	

NAME	H	Form Health Visitor
		DATE
Home/Surgery (insert H or S)		
Patient not Present		
New Baby Ist V.	CHILD	
General Health	CHILD	
Immunology	CHILD	
Con. re illness	CHILD	
Hearing test	CHILD	
Handicapped Ch.	CHILD	
A/N or P/N Adv.	I2-65	ADULT
Health problems	I2-65	ADULT
Obesity advice	I2-65	ADULT
Other advice	I2-65	ADULT
Health problems	Over 65	ADULT
Welfare or Social problems	Over 65	ADULT
Other advice	Over 65	ADULT
DIAGNOSIS IF APPOPRIATE		
OFFICE USE ONLY		

Table 1 Analysis of Consultations by Disease Groups

Disease group	Consultations at which this diagnosis was mentioned	Percentage of total consultations
Infective & parasitic	367	5.0
Malignant neoplasms	97	1.3
Benign neoplasms	14	0.2
Allergies etc.	283	3.9
Blood	148	2.0
Mental	1,048	14.4
Central nervous system	217	3.0
Eyes	215	2.9
Ears	317	4.3
Cerebro-vascular system	849	11.6
Respiratory system	1,813	24.8
Gastro-intestinal	587	8.0
Genito-urinary	428	5.9
Pregnancy	657	9.0
Skins	522	7.2
Loco-motor	585	8.0
Congenital anomaly	23	0.3
Perinatal	1	0.0
Symptoms etc.	56	0.8
Accidents etc.	392	5.4

Table 2 The Ten Most Frequent Diagnoses by Consultation

Diagnosis	Consultations at which this diagnosis was mentioned	% of total consultations
Upper respiratory tract infection	692	9.4
Depression (all types)	499	6.8
Ante-natal care	422	5.8
Acute bronchitis and bronchiolitis	309	4.2
Anxiety state	286	3.9
Congestive heart failure	231	3.2
Tonsillitis	190	2.6
Skin sepsis	178	2.4
Osteo-arthritis	175	2.4
Otitis media	142	2.0

Table 3 Multiple Diagnoses at Consultations

Number of diagnoses made	No. of consultations	Total	Percentage of consultations where that number of diagnoses was made
0	21	0	–
1	5,872	5,872	64.7
2	1,196	2,392	26.3
3	209	627	6.9
4	47	188	2.1
Total	7,345	9,079	100.0

Table 4 Diagnostic Referrals

	Total No.	Total abnormal	Percentage abnormal
Haematology (haemoglobin, erythrocyte sedimentation rate, white blood count etc (includes pregnancy haematology)	431	161	37
Bacteriology	335	168	50
Serology (inc. P.B.I., Rose-Waaler , pregnancy test)	120	36	30
Biochemistry	112	61	55
Histology (inc. smears)	88	26	30
Chest X-ray	41	16	39
Bone and joint X-ray	29	14	48
Barium meal X-ray	9	3	33
Gall bladder X-ray	9	7	78
I.V.P .	8	5	63
Other X-ray	6	5	83
Post-mortem	5	5	100
All types	1,193	507	43

Table 5 Number of Referrals to Out-Patient Departments per 1,000 Patients 1972

Patients in practice	Out-patient referrals	Referrals per 1,000 patients	Referrals per 1,000 patients England and Wales (hospital service statistics 1970)
3,137	201	64.1	171

Table 6 Number of Admissions per 1,000 patients 1972

Patients in practice	Admissions	Admissions per 1,000 patients	Admissions per 1,000 patients England and Wales (hospital service statistics 1970)
3,137	240	76.5	112.6

Table 7 Consultations per Patient in 1972

	Total	Males	Females
No of patients consulting	1,938	855	1,083
No on list	3,137	1,528	1,609
Percentage consulting	62	56	67
No of consultations	7,297	2,876	4,421
Average no of consultations per consulting patient	3.8	3.4	4.1
Average no of consultations per patient on list	2.3	1.9	2.7

Table 8 Attendances per Patient in 1972

	• Total	Males	Females
No of patients attending	1,825	812	1,013
No on list	3,137	1,528	1,609
Percentage attending	58	53	63
No of attendances	6,086	2,475	3,611
Average no of attendances per attending patient	3.3	3.0	3.6
Average no of attendances per patient on list	1.9	1.6	2.2

Table 9 Visits per Patient in 1972

	Total	Males	Females
No of patients visited	442	166	276
No on list	3,137	1,528	1,609
Percentage visited	14	11	17
No of visits	1,211	401	810
Average no of visits per visited patient	2.7	2.4	2.9
Average no of visits per patient on list	0.4	0.3	0.5

Table 10 Proportion of Households Contacted

Household size	No. of Households	Percentage contacted					
		Doctor			Nurse	HV	By doctor, nurse or HV
		Att.	Visit	Cons.			
1	751	44	11	47	12	1	48
2	300	80	25	82	30	9	82
3	177	93	27	93	38	18	95
4	146	94	37	95	47	26	96
5	69	100	41	100	57	28	100
6	28	96	46	100	68	18	100
7+	11	100	82	100	64	36	100

Table 11 Total Consultations by Age Group

Age group	0–1	1–4	5–9	10–14	15–44	45–64	65+	Total
Number consulting	52	139	192	149	766	358	282	1,938
Number on list	55	185	308	269	1,290	624	406	3,137
Percentage consulting	95	75	62	55	59	57	69	62
No of consultations	262	443	531	316	3,141	1,412	1,192	7,297
Av no of consultations per consulting patient	5.0	3.2	2.8	2.1	4.1	3.9	4.2	3.8
Av no of consultations per patient on list	4.8	2.4	1.7	1.2	2.4	2.3	2.9	2.3

Table 12 Total Attendances by Age Group

Age Group	0–1	1–4	5–9	10–14	15–44	45–64	65+	Total
Number attending	50	137	184	146	750	345	213	1,825
Number on list	55	185	308	269	1,290	624	406	3,137
Percentage attending	91	74	60	54	58	55	52	58
No. of attendances	221	391	493	297	2,825	1,167	692	6,086
Av no of attendances per attending patient	4.4	2.9	2.7	2.0	3.7	3.4	3.2	3.3
Av no of attendances per patient on list	4.0	2.1	1.6	1.1	2.2	1.9	1.7	1.9

Table 13 Total Visits by Age Group

Age group	0–1	1–4	5–9	10–14	15–44	45–64	65+	Total
Number visited	23	32	34	13	130	75	135	442
Number on list	55	185	308	269	1,290	624	406	3,137
Percentage visited	42	17	11	5	10	12	33	14
No of visits	41	52	38	19	316	245	500	1,211
Av no of visits per visited patient	1.8	1.6	1.1	1.5	2.4	3.3	3.7	2.7
Av no of visits per patient on list	0.7	0.3	0.1	0.1	0.2	0.4	1.2	0.4

Table 14 A/V Ratios by Age-Totals

Age group	No. of attendances	No. of visits	A/V ratio
0 - 4	612	93	6.6
5 - 9	493	38	13.0
10 - 14	297	19	15.6
15 - 44	2,825	316	8.9
45 - 64	1,167	245	4.8
65+	692	500	1.4
Total	6,086	1,211	5.0

Table 15 Total Consultations by Social Class

Social class	I & II	III	IV & V	Total
Number consulting	506	1,091	341	1,938
Number on list	812	1,740	585	3,137
Percentage consulting	62	63	58	62
No. of consultations	1,792	4,048	1,457	7,297
Av. no. of consultations per consulting patient	3.5	3.7	4.3	3.8
Av. no. of consultations per patient on list	2.2	2.3	2.5	2.3

Table 16 Total Attendances by Social Class

Social class	I & II	III	IV & V	Total
Number attending	486	1,035	304	1,825
Number on list	812	1,740	585	3,137
Percentage attending	60	60	52	58
No. of attendances	1,502	3,425	1,159	6,086
Av. no. of attendances per attending patient	3.1	3.3	3.8	3.3
Av. no of attendances per patient on list	1.8	2.0	2.0	1.9

Table 17 Total Visits by Social Class

Social Class	I & II	III	IV & V	Total
Number visited	100	242	100	442
Number on list	812	1,740	585	3,137
Percentage visited	12	14	17	14
Number of visits	290	623	298	1,211
Av. no. of visits per visited patient	2.9	2.6	3.0	2.7
Av. no. of visits per patient on list	0.4	0.4	0.5	0.4

Table 18 Social Class and Household Contact

Social class		I & II	III	IV & V	Total
No. of households		333	840	309	1,482
Doctor contact	%	73	68	64	68
Nurse contact	%	31	24	25	26
Health visitor contact	%	12	9	7	1
Contact with team	%	74	69	64	69

Table 19 A/V Ratios by Social Class-Totals

Social class	No. of attendances	No. of visits	A/V ratio
I & II	1,502	290	5.2
III	3,425	623	5.5
IV & V	1,159	298	3.9
Total	6,086	1,211	5.0

Table 20 Effect of Duration of Time on List on Consultation Rates

	No. of patients over 11 years in group	No. over 11 years never attended	Percentage over 11 years never attended	No. over 11 years never visited	Percentage over 11 years never visited	No. over 11 years never consulted	Percentage over 11 years never consulted
Registered 1970-1	458	173	38	381	83	142	31
Registered 1965-9	342	152	44	296	87	142	42
Registered 1960-5	417	180	43	372	89	170	41
Registered pre-1960	1,252	577	46	1,076	86	532	43

Table 21 A/V Ratio by Time on List-Totals

Time on list	Total attendances of patients over 11 years	Total visits of patients over 11 years	A/V ratio patients over 11 years
1970-1	1,031	253	4.1
1965-9	677	110	6.2
1960-4	810	99	8.2

Table 22 Patient-Initiated: Doctor-Initiated Consultations by Sex and Age Group

Age group	Male patient-initiated: doctor-initiated ratio	Female patient-initiated: doctor-initiated ratio	Total patient-initiated: doctor-initiated ratio
0-1	1:0.68	1:0.89	1:0.77
1-4	1:0.14	1:0.14	1:0.14
5-9	1:0.35	1:0.15	1:0.26
10-14	1:0.24	1:0.18	1:0.21
15-44	1:0.45	1:0.90	1:0.74
45-64	1:0.93	1:0.68	1:0.79
65+	1:1.06	1:0.81	1:0.9
Total	1:0.57	1:0.69	1:0.64

Table 23 Patient-Initiated: Doctor-Initiated Consultations by Sex and Social Class

	Male	Female	Total
	patient-initiated: doctor-initiated ratio	patient-initiated: doctor-initiated ratio	patient-initiated: patient-initiated ratio
I & II	1:0.52	1:0.71	1:0.63
III	1:0.53	1:0.66	1:0.61
IV & V	1:0.78	1:0.77	1:0.77
Total	1:0.57	1:0.69	1:0.64

Table 24 Consultation Workload and Proportion of Patients

Percentage of consultations	Percentage males causing this percentage of consultations	Percentage females causing this percentage of consultations	Percentage of total practice causing this percentage of consultations
100	56	67	62
90	38	45	42
75	25	30	27
50	12	15	13
25	4	6	5
10	2	5	4
5	< 2	< 5	< 4

Table 25 Surgery Attendance Workload and Proportion of Patients

Percentage of attendances	Percentage males causing this percentage of attendances	Percentage females causing this percentage of attendances	Percentage of total practice causing this percentage of attendances
100	53	63	58
90	25	43	40
75	24	28	26
50	12	14	13
25	4	5	5
10	1	3	2
5	< 1	< 3	< 2

Table 26 Visiting Workload and Proportion of Patients

Percentage of visits	Percentage of males causing this percentage of visits	Percentage females causing this percentage of visits	Percentage of total practice causing this percentage of visits
100	11	17	14
90	8	12	11
75	5	7	6
50	2	3	2
25	1	1	1
10	<1	1	1
5	<1	<1	<1

Table 27 Non-Consulters and High Consulters by Age Group – Totals

Age group	0-1	1-4	5-9	10-14	15-44	45-64	65+	Total
Percentage never attending	9	26	40	46	42	45	48	42
Percentage attending 6+ times	20	5	4	–	9	7	7	7
Percentage never visited	58	83	89	95	90	88	67	86
Percentage visited 6+ times	2	1	–	–	1	2	4	1
Percentage never consulted	6	25	38	45	41	43	31	38
Percentage consulted 6+ times	27	7	4	–	11	11	14	9

Table 28 Non-consulters and High Consulters by Social Class – Totals

Social class	1&2	3	4 & 5	Total
Percentage never attending	40	41	48	42
Percentage attending 6+ times	6	7	9	7
Percentage never visited	88	86	83	86
Percentage visited 6+ times	1	1	2	1
Percentage never consulted	38	38	42	38
Percentage consulted 6+ times	8	9	12	10

Table 29 Seasonal Variation of Consulting Rates

	Patient initiated			Doctor initiated			Total initiated		
	Attendances	Visits	Consultations	Attendances	Visits	Consultations	Attendances	Visits	Consultations
Spring	25	20	24	29	23	28	26	22	26
Summer	24	19	23	22	25	23	23	22	23
Autumn	26	23	26	25	27	25	26	25	26
Winter	25	38	27	25	25	25	25	30	26

Table 30 Attendances, Visits and Consultations by Day of Week

	No. of attendances	No. of visits	No. of consultations	Percentage of total consultations	A/V ratio
Monday	1,549	301	1,850	25	5.1
Tuesday	268	158	426	6	1.7
Wednesday	1,908	171	2,079	29	11.2
Thursday	970	216	1,186	16	4.5
Friday	1,271	182	1,453	20	7.0
Saturday	111	111	222	3	1.0
Sunday	9	72	81	1	0.1
Total	6,086	1,211	7,297	100	5.0

Table 31 Type of Nurse Consultation

	Surgery	Home	Total
New acute illness	205	103	308
Follow-up of acute illness	182	271	453
Follow-up of chronic illness	276	669	945
Post-hospital	7	147	154
Other	54	10	64
Total	724	1,200	1,924

Table 32 Follow-up Consultations by Nurse

Diagnosis	Surgery	Home	Total
'Senility'	0	174	174
Iron deficiency anaemia	118	50	168
Pernicious anaemia	49	103	152
Hypertension	57	12	99
C.H.F.	3	93	96
Varicose ulcer	3	79	82
Asthma	67	4	71
Cerebrovascular disease	0	40	40
Wax in ears	28	12	40
Chronic bronchitis	0	37	37
Tonsillitis	5	28	33
Coronary thrombosis	12	18	30
Osteo-arthritis	3	25	28
Multiple sclerosis	0	27	27
Pneumonia	5	22	27
Acute bronchitis	2	14	26
Hay fever	25	0	25
Minor injuries	11	13	24
Cellulitis	0	20	20
Cholecystitis	0	19	19
Rheumatoid arthritis	4	15	19

Table 33 Team Consultations 1972

	Attendances	Visits	A/V ratio	Consultation	Consultation per patient per annum
Doctor	6,086	1,211	5.0	7,297	2.3
Nurse	724	1,200	0.6	1,924	0.6
Health Visitor	493	74	6.7	567	0.2
Total	7,303	2,485	2.9	9,778	3.1

PART II THE PATIENT SATISFACTION SURVEY

8 THE SURVEY

Purpose

The purpose of the patient satisfaction survey was to ascertain the attitude and views of patients to the new style of primary health care described and discussed in Part I. This survey is also of general interest as the practice has the type of organisation and provides the team care which is becoming increasingly common and which will become the norm in practices operating from health centres. To accomplish the objects of the survey, questions which gave equal opportunity for favourable or unfavourable replies had to be asked about many aspects of health care. This could only be achieved by a survey which did not emanate from the team who provided the care which was to be commended or criticised. For the doctor, the nurses, the health visitor or the midwife to have asked the questions or to have been known to have instigated the survey and to have access to the replies would have inhibited the patients from expressing their views without fear or favour. It would thus have failed to elicit the maximum information and the freest expression of opinion.

In order to avoid this happening, the survey was conducted by the University of Durham, Department of Sociology and Social Administration under the direction of one of the authors. In this task, he had the encouragement and financial support of the research committee of the Newcastle-upon-Tyne Regional Hospital Board. It was agreed with the committee that reliable findings could be obtained by a questionnaire interview survey of a stratified random sample of the patients on the practice list.

The Questionnaire

Throughout the questionnaire were many questions orientating on areas where the doctor's workload had obviously been lowered by using other members of the team. There were several hypotheses to be tested:

First, that the patients were satisfied with the overall health care service they received.

Second, that they were satisfied with the care given by the individual members of the Primary Health Care Team.

Third, that patients prefer a personal doctor service albeit within the setting of the team.

Fourth, that patients clearly distinguished between the competence of qualified nurses and lay receptionists.

Fifth, that patients who had experienced a service would view it more favourably than those who were unfamiliar with it.

Sixth, that patients' satisfaction with the overall service and its components was unrelated to their age or social class.

Early drafts of the questionnaire were seen by all partners of the Norton practice and by the other members of the health care team. Most helpful comments were received from Professor Margot Jefferys. The interviewing team considered two drafts and suggested several improvements which were incorporated in the final version. A number of questions were tested individually and the final draft was revised on the basis of the experience of a small pilot survey. The questions were worded in colloquial terms so as to be comprehensible to people of all levels of intelligence.

The questionnaire enquired into satisfaction with seven aspects of health care – the practice premises (14 questions), the receptionists (16), the appointment system (11), the 'personal doctor' system (27), the doctor's method of work (9), the work of the nurse (27), and the work of the midwife and the health visitor (15). The interviewers were also asked to obtain as accurately as possible the occupation of the head of the household in which the respondent lived.

A special questionnaire was prepared for chronically ill housebound patients. This omitted the fifty-four questions which either presupposed familiarity with the practice premises and the staff working in them or were addressed to women with young children. Instead these patients were asked five additional questions and four others in modified form (nos.15,31,45,55) relating to their special status.

In the construction of the measurement scales for the questionnaire, a standard scheme was adhered to whenever possible. Questions enquiring about definite facts (have you ever received advice) or about facts showing a state of mind (would you mind getting advice) and requiring a yes/no option, always provided a third category of 'don't know'. Where the response of 'sometimes' was viable, this option appeared in the third position with 'don't know' in the fourth. For questions asking an opinion, a five-point scale was provided consisting of responses which ranged from very positive, positive, neutral, negative to very negative. Occasionally the order was reversed to guard against clustering. However, the scale always went from one extreme to the opposite one with ambivalence registering in the middle.

A five-point scale for the replies of a small subgroup, e.g. social class or age, will not give statistically significant results especially if the replies are fairly evenly distributed over all five cells. The larger the number of respondents in a cell, both absolutely and relatively to that of the subgroup, the more likely is it that the results will be statistically significant; that means, the greater will be the probability of differences in the replies being genuine and not the result of chance fluctuations due to sampling. Few subgroups and two-point scales maximise the number of findings which are significant but they simultaneously reduce the scope of respondents to express their views accurately and minimise the knowledge which can be derived from their replies. This diminishes the interest in a survey and the scope for action on the basis of its findings. The greater the divergence in the proportion of respondents giving different replies, e.g. 80 per cent very satisfied, 5 per cent very dissatisfied, the less important is the size of the subgroup.

In this survey as in most others, the size of the subgroup, e.g. the number of patients who had received a follow-up visit by the nurse, was not known in advance. The use of a five-point scale in questions leaves open the possibility of concentrating replies into a three or two-point scale, e.g. by combining 'satisfactory' with 'very satisfactory', when analysing and commenting on the replies.

The Sample

Children under the age of sixteen were not considered suitable respondents in an attitude survey and were therefore exluded. It would have been desirable, in some respects, to interview all adults on the doctor's list, but this would have been an expensive procedure in terms of money, effort and time, resulting in findings which in all probability would not have been markedly different from those of a stratified random sample. A comprehensive survey would have involved the interviewing of more than one member of a household in a large number of cases, a situation which might not have encouraged the veracity of replies.

The method of sampling adopted was to divide the adult population into five categories of users: (1) chronic housebound, (2) recipients of intensive care, (3) the nurse – first users, (4) the minimal users and (5) the normal users. Each of these categories was composed of users who on account of their different experiences might have had distinct attitudes to the primary health care service or to some of its components.

Patients were categorised as chronic housebound if they were permanently on the doctor's visiting list and likely to remain so in the foreseeable future. All in this category were to be interviewed. The 'intensive care' category was defined as those patients who, in 1972, had seen the doctor twice in one day on at least one occasion or three times in at least one week or five times in at least one month. One third of this category were selected for interview. The 'nurse-first' users were those patients, excluding recipients of intensive care and minimal users, who, in 1972, had asked for a visit by the doctor but instead had been visited by the nurse. All in this category were to be interviewed. Minimal users were all those who, in 1972, had either not seen the doctor at all or had seen him only once. One in fourteen of this category were selected for interview.

The remaining names on the doctor's list were described as normal users. The sampling fraction applied to each age and sex group of this category reflected the extent to which they used the service. For the youngest age group (16-19 years) disproportionately more had to be selected in order to obtain a minimum for each cell. This method of sampling resulted in 60 per cent of those selected being female. That in fact equalled the proportion of female consultations, as was shown in the doctor's workload survey. About one in four of all normal users were selected for interview.

The data required for the selection of the sample were obtained from the computer print-outs which had been compiled for the workload survey. The sheets gave for each patient on the doctor's list the name, age, sex, category of user and the number of consultations with the doctor in 1972. The addresses of the patients selected were abstracted from the surgery record cards. The aggregate number in the sample was 417 – 20 per cent of the adult patients on the doctor's list.

The Interview

In any survey, the endeavour to produce findings which accurately reflect the attitude of the population sampled is beset with many difficulties. Some of these can be overcome by the use of well-established techniques which however are not dogmatic rules but require expertise in their application as well as considerable familiarity with the subject matter of the survey. Such techniques help in determining the appropriate size of a sample, in the proper selection of a sample, in the design of a questionnaire, in the training of interviewers and in the editing and processing of the completed questionnaires.

The appearance, manners, social class, sex, language, accent and other characteristics of interviewers will also, to a greater or lesser extent, affect the genuineness of a respondent's answers. The respondent's perception, if any, of the organisation conducting the survey and the avowed and suspected purpose of the survey are other factors which, at least in certain circumstances, will affect the nature of the response. About these important aspects of interviewing as well as about many others, there are no well-established techniques to assist the researcher.

In this survey it was considered important to stresss the independence and respectability of the organisation conducting the survey, its public service object and the confidentiality of the replies given. It was, however, also important to avoid the suspicion that the survey was prying on the doctor or the other members of the health care team. To achieve these objectives, a number of measures were taken. The persons selected for interview were sent a letter which is reproduced on page 118 three days before the interviewer called on them. This letter explained the nature and aims of the survey and emphasised its link with the university by the notepaper heading and by referring to the interviewers as senior members of the university or its colleges.

It also made quite clear that the doctor was not merely cognisant of the questions which were to be asked but positively approved and hoped that his patients would assist. The letter also contained a categorical and authoritative assurance that the replies would be confidential to the university staff and would not be seen by the doctor.

The interviews were conducted at the respondents' homes between 21 February and 14 March 1973 by a team of eleven interviewers, all of whom were closely associated with the university – two were postgraduate students, three ordinands, two former social workers, one a non-practising medical doctor, one a former health visitor and two personal tutors to students. All the interviewers were resident in Durham city some twenty miles from Norton so that it was virtually certain that none of them would be known even by sight to the respondents. Most of them were known to the director of the survey as persons of maturity, discretion and tact and all of them were familiar with the objects of the survey.

The interviewers were selected partly for their personal characteristics and partly to confirm in the respondent's mind the link between the survey and the university. All of them were highly educated and most of them were in speech, appearance and manners quite distinctly social class I. Whether and, if so, to what extent and in what direction this influenced the nature of the responses is not known, but it is a possibility which should be kept in mind.

The duration of the interviews varied widely and ranged from about half an hour to one and a half hours. It was felt that they were long enough to allay anxiety and dispel any efforts by the patient to gloss over his problems.

Certain factual questions about the premises, and the patient's method of getting there, were purposely put first in order to disarm the patient and establish rapport. Several of the interviewers reported difficulties among older respondents in concentrating for such long periods. Others experienced difficulties in interviewing the respondent on his/her own. This meant that occasionally the replies, while made by the respondent, reflected the attitude of a more dominant member of the household.

Up to three calls were made at the respondent's address to obtain an interview. The final response rate was 82 per cent, a reasonably satisfactory proportion. Among the categories, as was to be expected, it was least (67 per cent) for the minimal users but was above 78 per cent for the other four categories. Among normal users it was 79 per cent for males and 85 per cent for females and was least (74 per cent) for the lowest age group. Very few people refused to be interviewed but quite a few had moved while others could not be interviewed because of their state of health. There is no reason to suspect that the respondents interviewed are not representative of the sample selected.

The Analysis of the Questionnaires

To each questionnaire, a sheet was attached giving data about the respondents which were abstracted from the computer off-prints of the workload survey. These included the category of user, age and sex. To this was added social class based on the occupation of heads of households which had been ascertained in the interviews. The workload survey had made use of the standard classification of the Registrar General which has five social classes. The disadvantage of this classification is that class III contains more than half the population and consists of both manual and white-collar workers. For the purpose of the patient satisfaction survey an analysis by four social classes was considered more meaningful:

I Professional, managerial and skilled white-collar workers.
II Routine white-collar workers.
III Skilled manual workers.
IV Semi-skilled and unskilled manual workers.

In this classification, I is the same as the first two classes of the Registrar General, IV is the same as his last two classes while II and III comprise his large intermediate class.

The analysis of social and medical data by class is as important as it is difficult and subject to pitfalls. Many wives and adult children have occupations falling into a classification different from that of the head of the household. Respondents frequently do not know the occupation of their husband or father sufficiently accurately for correct classification. Some respondents are reluctant to give their occupation as it seems to them irrelevant, while others give it inaccurately in order to upgrade their social status. The distinction between various degrees of skill among manual workers, the borderline between skilled and routine white-collar workers and even the difference between manual and non-manual workers are in quite a number of cases somewhat arbitrary. In this survey, for all but one respondent, a social classification could be made and all were made as accurately as the evidence available permitted.

The questionnaire had been designed so that the replies and the data giving age, sex, social class and category of user could be punched on to computer cards without having to be transcribed on to any other records. In retrospect it appears that the editing of the questionnaire was not perfect. This is shown by some slight inconsistencies in the analysis of the results reproduced in the Appendix. In no case has this led to any significant distortion of the results.

The analysis of the data was made by the Durham University computer using the University of Michigan statistical package for the social sciences' Crostabs with Statistics programme. The replies to the questions were aggregated and classified by five user categories, five age groups and four social classes. The computer calculated for each question the three chi square significances of the percentage analyses.

On account of the method of selecting the sample the proportion of respondents giving a particular answer was not representative of all the patients in the practice. In order to give an approximate representation of the attitude of all patients the replies for each age-sex group of normal users and for each of the other four categories were grossed-up. This was done by multiplying the replies to each question by the aggregate number of patients in the age-sex group or category of the respondent and dividing by the corresponding number of respondents: for example, the reply of a female normal user aged 20-34 was multiplied by 120 and divided by 41, a grossing factor of 2.93; a reply by a minimal user was multiplied by 1,108 and divided by 50, a grossing factor of 22.16. This is a sound method of estimating the attitude of all patients but as the fifty minimal user respondents represented just over half of all the adult patients in the practice, the estimate is very approximate. The confidence which can be placed in the estimates is however greater than the small number of minimal user respondents indicates, as the differences in replies between respondents in the various categories, age groups and social classes to most questions are relatively small.

All respondents who gave negative replies to certain questions (nos 16, 17, 19, 20, 41, 53, 57, 58, 59, 61, 63, 70, 72, 85, 86, 91 and 94) were listed and a table was compiled showing for each respondent the questions to which he had replied negatively. This made it possible to distinguish respondents who were negative all round from those who were negative in respect of one component of the service or negative in reply to only one question. The number of respondents who answered the questions relating to the work of the midwife (32) and the health visitor (39,43) was too small to obtain meaningful results from an analysis by category, age and social class. The same was the case for the twenty-five chronic housebound respondents. The questions relating to these two sections of the questionnaire are reproduced but not the actual figures. A summary of the findings is however given in the next chapter.

The Respondents

The sample contained five categories of users. Three of these – the chronic housebound, recipients of 'intensive care' and 'nurse-first' users – were composed of patients whose attitude was specially relevant to the purpose of the survey; a fourth whose size was quite arbitrarily determined was made up of minimal users who were thought to be least familiar with the service; the fifth group, consisting of the remainder, was weighted by sex and age so as to represent broadly the use made of the service. The response rates for the various categories were sufficiently similar for the respondents to be representative of the sample selected but, as has already been pointed out, they were by no means representative of the patients on the practice list. Thus, females accounted for just over half the adults on the list but nearly two thirds of the sample. This is explained by the predominance of females among the chronic housebound (many of whom were very old) the nurse-first users (many of whom had young children) and the normal users (women make more use of the service). When the grossing-up factors were applied to the respondents, the resulting patient population had a sex ratio very close to that of the adult list. This was brought about mainly because the minimal user respondents were, in this respect, representative of all patients in this category.

The composition of respondents by category of user was in the nature of the sample quite different from that of the patients on the practice list. Thus, over 50 per cent of all adults on the practice list but only 15 per cent of the respondents were minimal users. The age distribution of the sample was equally unrepresentative, the under 35s and the over 65s being over-represented while the middle-aged were under-represented.

University of Durham Department of Sociology and Social Administration

44 Old Elvet, Durham DH1 3JQ

PATIENT SATISFACTION SURVEY

Telephone: Durham 4466 (STD code 0385)

____

Dear

We are conducting a survey to find out what patients think about the services they receive from their general practitioners. The object of the survey is to look for ways of improving the standards of care patients receive.

A group of patients from your doctor's list has been selected by the University team to be interviewed as part of this survey. Your name has come up amongst that group.

Your doctor knows about this survey and has seen the questions we would like to put to you. He welcomes this study and hopes that you will assist us. The information you give us will be treated in the strictest confidence. The University team will not let the doctor know the answers given by any individual patient. The question forms will not be seen by anyone but the members of the University conducting the survey.

It is only through the participation of a cross section of *all* the people who use the services that it will be possible to find out how to improve them, so even if you feel that, because you are satisfied with the services, you have no comments to make, it is very important to the success of the study that we have your answers to our questions. We would, therefore, be most grateful for your help.

All the interviewers are senior members of the University or it's colleges. I have arranged for ________

________________ to call at your home on ________ the ________

of ________________ in the morning/afternoon/evening.

She/he will have a letter of identification.

Yours faithfully,

P.R. Kaim-Caudle

P.R. Kaim-Caudle
Senior Lecturer in
Social Administration
Director of the Patient
Satisfaction Survey Team

9 THE FINDINGS

Summary

This chapter gives the findings of the survey; comments on them are made in the next chapter. In spite of the small size of the sample the major findings are quite definite and not subject to any but the most improbable sampling error.

The overwhelming majority of respondents (95 per cent or more), irrespective of age and social class who expressed an opinion, assessed the practice premises as good or excellent, considered that the receptionists gave an average or good service, were satisfied or very satisfied with the overall treatment they received from the doctor, considered him as concerned or very concerned with the patient's problem, approved both treatment by a nurse at the surgery after they had seen the doctor and follow-up visits by her after an initial visit by the doctor and assessed the health visitor's well-baby clinic as well organised and her immunisation clinics as helpful or very helpful.

In spite of these very positive general findings there were undoubted objections by a substantial minority of respondents to certain conduct and procedures. These negative responses were usually made in reply to specific questions. Twenty-five per cent or more did or would object at least sometimes to telling the receptionist at the surgery why they wanted to see the doctor, to her enquiring about treatment from the doctor or to her passing on a message from the doctor about the result of clinical tests. A similar proportion felt that they had usually to wait a long time on keeping an appointment to see the doctor and over half of these were annoyed or very annoyed about having to do so. A third to whom the question applied felt that the doctor would not always let them have a certificate of incapacity to work when they needed it. A visit by the nurse when one by the doctors had been requested was thought unsatisfactory by a quarter of those who had this experience but by half of those who did not.

A substantial minority of the small number of women who had received ante-natal care would have been unhappy to receive routine care from the midwife.

The first, second, third, fourth and sixth hypotheses which the replies to the questionnaire were to test, were found valid beyond any reasonable doubt, while the fifth was not proved conclusively but the replies indicate that it is probably valid.

In the detailed findings given in the following sections, the phraseology used is that of the questionnaire. This colloquial language conveys the views of respondents better than an account in more academic terminology.

The Tables contain an analysis of the replies to the first 101 questions by the five categories of users, the five age groups and the four social classes. In this chapter, reference to this analysis is made only when the differences between categories, groups and classes are statistically significant (see notes on the Tables) by the chi square test calculated by the computer which did the analysis. To the great majority of questions, the differences in replies are too small to be significant. This was more often due to the uniformity of response than to the small size of the subgroups.

The Premises

This section was concerned with ascertaining facts relating to the number of persons attending the surgery, the nature of the difficulties, if any, experienced in getting there and the number who had received attention in the nurse's treatment room. Opinions were asked about the standard of the premises and of the nurse's treatment room and enquiries made about any changes which were desirable with regard to the waiting room.

About seven in ten of all adults and nine in ten of the sample, excluding the chronic housebound patients, had attended the surgery in the past year. One in ten had experienced difficulty in getting there. The two most common causes were long journey (11) and transportation problems (17). Only five respondents referred to medical conditions, two to difficult working hours and one to small children at home. Among the 39 reasons given, 32 came from the 176 respondents from social classes III and IV (manual workers) and only 7 from the 139 respondents in classes I and II.

Not a single person considered the practice premises as poor or very poor while almost all considered them as excellent or good.

About one in eight of the sample would have liked to see some changes in the waiting room. Most of the suggestions were reasonable, practicable and would not involve any great expense. The list of suggestions included a fish tank, greater variety of current magazines, plants, music and more comfortable chairs. There were also several suggestions to permit smoking!

About half of the respondents had received attention in the nurse's treatment room. None considered this room as poorly or very poorly equipped while five out of six took the opposite view.

The Receptionists

This section elicited views on the behaviour and attitude of receptionists, asked for an assessment of the quality of the service they rendered, enquired into the extent to which patients objected, in different situations, to communicating with the doctor either through a receptionist or a qualified nurse and asked about the willingness of patients to receive advice about their health from either a receptionist or a qualified nurse.

Nine in ten of the respondents and about the same proportion of all adult patients had spoken to the receptionists at some time. The majority who had not done so were among the chronic housebound and the minimal users. This explains why the over 65s and the under 20s had least contact with the receptionists.

Overt criticism of the personalities and attitudes of receptionists was fairly rare: only 2 per cent of respondents considered them very unpleasant or unpleasant, only 3 per cent very unhelpful or unhelpful and 4 per cent attributed to them a couldn't-care-less attitude. Two thirds thought them concerned or very concerned about patients while one sixth considered them as unconcerned. Comments recorded by interviewers make it doubtful whether unconcern indicated an absence of need for concern or whether it referred to an indifferent attitude. These opinions relate to four receptionists collectively. Remarks made by the respondents make it appear that one was less liked than the others.

Some 8 per cent of the sample felt that the receptionists usually or always rushed them. This feeling was most marked with the younger age groups. Three quarters thought that receptionists were helping them to see the doctor – a view more widely held by older patients and probably also by social class IV (unskilled).

The general attitude of respondents to receptionists appears slightly ambiguous. Only 1 per cent rated the receptionists' service poor; 96 per cent rated it average or good. However, forty-eight individual respondents, about 16 per cent of those who were asked these questions, gave a negative reply to at least one of the four questions referring to pleasantness, helpfulness, rushing or making it difficult to see the doctor. This discrepancy between the general rating and the assessment of specific characteristics may be more apparent than real. It is quite reasonable to feel that a woman is unpleasant or unhelpful or rushes you and yet consider that all in all she renders an average or good service.

An appreciable proportion of respondents had a different attitude to receptionists than to qualified nurses. Only 8 per cent minded or minded sometimes telling a nurse at the surgery why they wanted to see the doctor but the corresponding proportion for a receptionists was 30 per cent. The reluctance to tell the receptionist was greater among the younger than the older age groups. The proportion who minded or minded sometimes telling a receptionist why they wanted a visit from the doctor was lower (16 per cent). Here too, reluctance declined with age. A mere 5 per cent minded or minded sometimes telling a nurse why they wanted a visit.

Just over 25 per cent of respondents objected or objected sometimes to the receptionist giving them a message from the doctor relating to clinical tests. This objection was greatest among minimal and nurse-first users and also among the very young and those in late middle age. The proportion of respondents who minded or sometimes minded the receptionist enquiring from the doctor about some treatment for them was about 30 per cent; this too was greatest among minimal and nurse-first users, and was also decidedly greater for white-collar than for manual workers. Three quarters of respondents would mind receiving advice about their health from a receptionist. The objection to this was least among the over 65s.

About a fifth of normal users, three quarters of the chronic housebound but only a tenth of the minimal users had at some time received advice about their health from a nurse. About 16 per cent of all respondents did mind or would sometimes mind receiving such advice. The objection would be least among the young and the old.

The Appointment System

In this section respondents were asked how they made appointments to see the doctor, whether they liked an appointment system, what difficulty, if any, they experienced in seeing a doctor in different circumstances, whether they had to wait long on keeping an appointment and, if so, what was their reaction to being kept waiting.

Five out of six of all patients on the doctor's list made the appointment to see the doctor by phone; nearly half used their own phone, three out of ten used a public phone and the remainder had someone else make the call. About one in eight called at the surgery to make an appointment. The proportion of patients in the sample making telephone appointments was almost the same but fewer used their own phone and more had someone else make the call. The replies to the method of appointment question showed greater differences for all three classifications – category of user, age groups and social class – than those to any other question. The differences however are much as was to be expected. Thus, more than half of the chronic sick had someone else make a call and only a quarter used their own phone. The lowest and the highest age groups had least access to private phones, many more of the over 65s – one fifth – than of the other age groups called at the surgery for an appointment, fewer of them used a public phone and as many as three in ten had someone else make a call. The proportion of patients using their own phone had the expected class gradient varying from 77 to 21 per cent and inversely for a public phone varying from 9 to 39 per cent.

These very substantial differences in the convenience of making an appointment make it all the more astonishing that more than nine in ten of all respondents expressed satisfaction with the doctor having an appointment system and that this high rate of approval was shared by all categories of users, age groups and social classes.

About a quarter of all patients and slightly more of the sample had at some time difficulty in seeing their doctor. The nurse-first users experienced more frequent difficulties than other categories and so did the young adults, while the old had least difficulty.

As many as three in five had at one time wished to see the doctor urgently, meaning the same day. The proportion who did so was decidedly greater among the chronic housebound, the intensive care and the nurse-first patients than among the normal and minimal user categories. In this urgent situation, a quarter could not see their own doctor and one in eight could only see him sometimes. About 6 per cent of the respondents who wanted to see their doctor urgently were seen neither by him nor by one of his partners but by a nurse. Among those ten patients, four felt that their health had suffered as a result of not seeing a doctor.

About one in six of the sample objected at least sometimes to explaining to the receptionists the reason for the urgency. This objection was strongest among the nurse-first users.

One in six of all patients but nearly a quarter of the sample usually had to wait a long time on keeping an appointment to see the doctor. (This phrase was not defined.) The proportion was highest among teenagers and declined for each age group in a remarkably regular pattern – from 41 to 8 per cent. Among those who had to wait, half expressed themselves as annoyed or very annoyed. This feeling was most pronounced among the nurse-first and minimal users.

It is interesting to note that among the thirty-seven annoyed respondents, fifteen were also critical of some aspect of the receptionist's service and seventeen of some aspect of the personal doctor system. As many as twelve of them gave critical answers to questions in at least two other sections of the questionnaire while eleven expressed annoyance at having to wait but were not critical of any other aspect.

The Personal Doctor System

This section dealt with the extent of patient attachment to their doctor and the reasons for it; enquired whether female patients preferred a woman doctor; solicited an overall assessment of the treatment patients received from the doctor and asked specific questions requiring an expression of opinion about particular aspects of patient-doctor contacts and relations.

More than nine out of ten respondents were aware that each doctor in the practice had his own list of patients. Nearly five out of six preferred to see their own doctor at the surgery. This wish was least among teenagers and was probably slightly less for all ages in respect of home visits. Virtually all respondents who preferred to see their own doctor felt that he knew and understood them, about two thirds felt they knew and understood him, only a fifth thought he was better than the other doctors, and a few made the point that he was more conversant with their past history.

About a fifth of all female patients and one sixth of female respondents would like to consult a woman doctor at least sometimes. This preference was most frequent with teenagers and least with young adults.

The most crucial question asked of respondents was: 'As for the treatment you receive from the doctor in general would you say you were . . . .' to this 49 per cent replied very satisfied, 43 per cent satisfied, 6 per cent did not know or had mixed feelings and 2 per cent were dissatisfied or very dissatisfied. (Only one respondent was in the latter category). The least favourable responses came from the minimal users, some of whom had not consulted the doctor for a year or more and gave a don't know answer. In spite of this high level of satisfaction with the general treatment they received, respondents were quite critical in their replies to specific questions.

About six out of seven felt able to consult the doctor about more than one condition at any one attendance and four out of five felt able to talk to him about problems or difficulties which were not medical. Several respondents felt that non-medical problems were not a doctor's concern and others thought he had enough to do with curing people who were ill.

Ninety per cent of patients felt that the doctor always or often gave them sufficient time and did not hurry them while only 6 per cent felt that he did so seldom or never. Only 6 per cent felt that their doctor did not give them a thorough examination when necessary. An even smaller fraction thought that the doctor's referrals to hospital were either excessive or insufficient.

A remarkably high number of respondents felt that the doctor did not or sometimes did not let them have a certificate of incapacity to work when they needed one; three out of five stated that this question did not apply to them and of the remainder, one third (forty-five respondents) gave a negative reply. For the 35-49 age group this proportion was about half. The social class differences in replies were too small to be statistically significant.

Almost all the sample felt that the doctor prescribed medicines neither too readily nor not often enough.

The great majority of respondents felt that the doctor explained things to them fully and answered all their questions, but 5 per cent replied negatively to the question soliciting this information and a further 7 per cent responded with sometimes.

Replies to a more general question about the doctor's concern for the patient were also overwhelmingly favourable. As many as 92 per cent considered him concerned or very concerned about their problems while only 3 per cent considered him unconcerned and a mere two patients thought he could not care less.

In an appreciable proportion of households not all members had the same doctor. About one in eight of respondents formed single-person households. This category included two fifths of the over 65s and of the chronic housebound. In one quarter of the two or more person-households, not all members had the same doctor. This proportion varied noticeably by social class – 11, 24, 29, 33 per cent (un-skilled). Four out of five respondents living in households where all members had the same doctor felt they had a 'family doctor' – a term which was not defined.

The pattern of replies in this section is in an important respect very similar to that in the section about receptionists. The proportion of negative responses to general questions was small and the positive responses overwhelmingly great. This was the case both to the question about satisfaction with the general treatment received, which was asked before the specific questions, and to the question about the doctor's concern which was asked after these questions. However, the number of individual respondents who made a negative reply, excluding sometimes, to at least one of the four questions relating to insufficient time, thorough examination, necessary tests, explaining fully, was fifty-five, that is 16 per cent of all respondents. A further twenty-four respondents gave a critical response only to the question relating to certification for incapacity to work.

Among the fifty-five who responded negatively to at least one of the four questions, fourteen were also annoyed about having to wait on keeping an appointment with the doctor, nine were critical about some aspect of the doctor's method of work and eight about some aspect of the nurses' work. In aggregate, thirteen of them gave a critical answer to questions in at least two other sections while twenty-two were critical only in response to questions about the personal doctor system.

The Doctor's Method of Working

This brief section contained questions relating to home visits by the doctor and to the consequences of the doctor's conduct on the patients' health; it also enquired into the extent to which patients phone the doctor for advice.

About one in six respondents felt that the doctor was reluctant to visit them at home; this proportion increased to nearly one in four when those who considered him sometimes reluctant are included. Forty per cent of the patients on whom the nurse called first had this feeling which was also probably more frequent among the younger than the older age groups. One in five of those who considered him reluctant (ten respondents) thought that their health had suffered as a result.

One in four of all respondents, excluding the chronic housebound, had struggled to the surgery at some time when they would have preferred a home visit by the doctor; seven of these respondents felt that their health had suffered as a result.

In all, thirteen individual respondents felt that their health had suffered either on account of the doctor's reluctance to visit or because they had struggled to the surgery. Four of these felt their health had suffered for both these reasons, another six had given negative responses to questions in at least two other sections while two had not given a negative response to any other question.

More than one in four respondents, excluding the chronic housebound, had telephoned the doctor for advice at some time. This proportion, as was to be expected, was least for the minimal users (8 per cent) and was also only 10 per cent for the two age groups over fifty. The two higher social classes probably sought more telephonic advice, but the evidence on this is inconclusive.

The Nurses

In this section respondents were asked whether they had received services from nurses in certain circumstances – at the surgery, first call on patient, follow-up visits – and, if so, whether these had been satisfactory. Respondents who had not received such services were asked how they would have reacted to them in the same circumstances.

About four fifths of respondents, excluding the chronic housebound, knew that qualified nurses worked from the doctor's surgery; the corresponding proportion was one half for the health visitor and somewhat lower for the midwife. This knowledge was least among minimal users and teenagers, and for the health visitor and the midwife was especially high in the 20-35 age group. Relatively few respondents knew about social workers or marriage guidance counsellors working from the surgery.

Almost half of all respondents had received treatment from a nurse in the surgery after they had seen the doctor. Very few patients (6 per cent) who had had such treatment would have preferred to have received it from the doctor. An even smaller number were opposed to nurses doing that sort of job for the doctor. However, objection against the nurse instead of the doctor treating minor complaints in the surgery was more common; almost one in five held this view.

More than one in five respondents or their children, excluding the chronic housebound, but approximately only one in ten of all patients had been visited by a nurse when in fact they had sent for the doctor. Seventy-five per cent of those who had received such visits were satisfied with the advice and treatment they had received from the nurse but all the same more than half would have preferred a visit from the doctor. The differences by age group or social class of those who were dissatisfied with the nurse's visit were too small to be statistically significant. About one in six who had received such visits (twelve patients) felt that their health had suffered because the nurse called rather than the doctor.

Twenty respondents, three out of ten, felt either that the nurse's treatment and advice had been unsatisfactory or that their health had suffered as a result of the nurse calling instead of the doctor. Eight of these felt that the visit from the nurse had been unsatisfactory but did not feel that their health had suffered. Eight of the twenty had given negative or critical replies to questions in at least two other sections.

Those respondents who had not been visited by a nurse when they had sent for the doctor were asked if they would mind if this were to happen. To this almost half replied that they would not mind and another 12 per cent replied that they would mind sometimes. Thus there seems little doubt that the objection against this procedure was greater among those who had not experienced it than among those who had.

One in three respondents or their children, including the chronic housebound, had been visited by a nurse at home as a follow-up of the doctor's visit. Almost all of them considered the advice and treatment they had received from the nurse satisfactory. With only very few exceptions they also felt confident that the nurse would report any new problems to the doctor and that he would take the necessary action. Only two patients, both in the nurse-first category, felt that their health had suffered as a result of such a follow-up visit. All the same, about a quarter of respondents would have preferred a follow-up visit from the doctor.

Those patients who had not received a follow-up visit from a nurse were asked if they would mind if this were to happen. Only 4 per cent replied that they would and the same proportion replied that they would sometimes mind. Very few of these respondents (2 per cent) lacked confidence in the nurse reporting new problems to the doctor or in the doctor taking the necessary action. The answers to these questions indicate that the objections against follow-up visits by the nurse are very few and are much the same irrespective of whether respondents did or did not experience such a visit.

The findings of this section appear to be fairly definite. Objections against the nurse treating patients in the surgery after they have seen the doctor and against a visit from the nurse following up one made by the doctor are fairly minimal. A considerable proportion of respondents, although markedly fewer than 50 per cent, objected to the nurse rather than the doctor treating minor complaints in the surgery and to a nurse making a visit when one by the doctor had been requested.

The Health Visitor and the Midwife

Half of the sixty women respondents who had children under the age of seven had attended the surgery for ante-natal care during the previous three years. About half of these had at some time been seen by the midwife without the doctor being present. The great majority of those who had that experience felt that the midwife did the same job as the doctor. However, a substantial minority of all women respondents who had received ante-natal care would have been unhappy or very unhappy if the midwife provided the routine care with the doctor seeing them only occasionally or in case of any abnormality.

About half of the women with children under seven had attended the well-baby clinic at the surgery. Most of them had attended regularly and virtually all thought the clinic was well organised. The great majority found the advice received from the health visitor helpful. The immunisation clinic organised by the health visitor was generally considered helpful by the great majority of the rather larger number of respondent mothers who attended it. Some half of the mothers with children under seven had at some time received advice about their children's health problems from the health visitor. This had been acceptable to most of them. About half of the mothers have had or would seek advice from the health visitor when their children were not well. All of them did or would have thought it acceptable.

Chronic Housebound Patients

The nurse from time to time called in place of the doctor on twenty-one out of the twenty-five chronic housebound patients. Fourteen of these patients thought that the doctor and the nurse did the same job when they saw them; one thought that her health had suffered as a result of the nurse rather than the doctor visiting her. All but one of the patients visited by the nurse felt confident that she would report any new problems they might have back to the doctor and were equally confident that the doctor would take the necessary action.

10 COMMENTS AND CONCLUSIONS

Findings – Not Facts

The purpose of the survey was to ascertain the attitude and views of patients to the new style of Primary Health Care described in Part I. The replies reflect the memory, perceptions and opinions of patients, they are not necessarily correct in any other respect. Thus the number of patients who said they had been to the surgery during the past year was based on memory which may well have been faulty and therefore may disagree with the records kept at the centre. The difficulties in getting to the surgery were those which the respondents perceived and were not necessarily the same as those which would appear reasonable to an unprejudiced outsider. The respondents were asked to pronounce on the equipment of the nurse's treatment room. Here again, their views were subjective and not based on expert knowledge; a medically qualified assessor might well have expressed quite a different opinion. An affirmative reply to the question, 'Do the receptionists rush you?' is not conclusive evidence that the patients were rushed but a valid statement that they felt they were rushed. The five questions enquiring whether a patient's health suffered in certain circumstances did not and could not possibly elicit a fact but really asked for an expression of opinion. In any case, the phrase 'suffered' was left intentionally vague. It might have referred to a permanent ill effect or merely to some slight temporary discomfort or some brief increase in the duration of an illness.

Similarly, an opinion that the treatment or advice received from a nurse was unsatisfactory was the patient's perception, not a professional assessment of the nurse's competence. The finding that well over 90 per cent of respondents were satisfied or very satisfied with the treatment they received from the doctor is very important but does not of course justify the conclusion that the treatment was satisfactory. The respondents were not able to assess properly the quality of the treatment they received nor the quantity they required. A dissatisfied patient of one doctor may have received better care than the satisfied patients of the same or another doctor. The findings however do demonstrate that the type of primary health care practised at Norton was felt to be satisfactory by the great majority of patients.

Findings of an Employee Satisfaction Survey

It is interesting and relevant to compare the findings of the survey with other attempts to measure satisfaction. In a study[1] undertaken by Opinion Research Centre in November 1974 (based on a systematic probability sample of 2083 full-time workers in private companies of twenty or more employees in one hundred constituencies throughout Great Britain), the question was asked: 'Overall, how satisfied are you with the terms and conditions of your job?' To this, 85 per cent replied fairly satisfied or very satisfied while only 8 per cent gave the contrary reply. However, nearly one in two workers thought they did not get a fair share of the cake they helped to provide and 23 per cent were dissatisfied with the way in which their employer kept them informed about important decisions and events which affected them personally. The pattern here appears to be similar to that found in our survey – a feeling of very widespread overall satisfaction is quite compatible with an expression of dissatisfaction by a substantial minority on specific but important issues.

False Conclusions

One of the noteworthy findings is that a visit by the nurse when one by the doctor had been requested was thought unsatisfactory by 25 per cent of the respondents who had this experience and by 50 per cent who had not. This should not be considered as a conclusive argument that such visits are harmful to the health of the patient or incompatible with good modern health care practice. Many people have a preference for the familiar and are apprehensive about innovations. Such an attitude naturally leads to a feeling of dissatisfaction when encountering a new situation. This general feeling is possibly accentuated when a familiar figure who is felt by the great majority of patients to know and understand them is replaced by a less familiar figure. Moreover the majority of patients who saw the nurse when they had requested the doctor were thinking usually of one particular occasion. It is quite possible that their satisfaction with doctor care on that occasion would not have been totally favourable either. An earlier chapter refers to the importance of nurse training and it would seem possible that if nurses were carefully instructed in the primary care of carefully selected new home visits they could considerably increase the level of satisfaction. This would be even more enchanced if the patients were made aware that the nurse had had special training.

In a health care system which is free at the point of consumption, there is a perfectly natural tendency for the patient, as consumer, to prefer what appears to him the best service irrespective of implications related to cost, efficiency and manpower shortage. If patients in a surgical ward were asked whether they would prefer to be operated on by the consultant or by a less experienced, less well qualified junior surgeon, there is little doubt as to the preference of the great majority. It is however very doubtful whether in cases of relatively straightforward operations, the patient's health is detrimentally affected by operations being performed by junior surgeons. In this example, the preference of the majority of patients would be perfectly reasonable and, in the rare case when something unforeseen happens, would be clearly to their advantage, but all the same, patients' preferences – free choice of surgeon – are clearly incompatible with the provision of a universal and comprehensive health service.

Some Tentative Comments

In medical care, the patient's state of mind and, in particular, his confidence in those who advise and treat him, are themselves often important factors in the cure of a disease. In this context, the dissatisfaction of a sizeable minority of patients with some aspect of the service indicates a situation which ought to be remedied whenever possible. Unfortunately in some instances no remedy is available.

Dissatisfaction with the health care service may be a manifestation of transference of dissatisfaction from some quite unrelated condition, for example, at work or within the family. In other instances, the patient's grievance about not being cured of asthma, chronic bronchitis, rheumatoid arthritis or similar diseases may manifest itself in dissatisfaction with the service, as the patient is unaware of the limitations of medical science.

Another cause of patient dissatisfaction is an unfamiliar situation which has arisen for reasons which he does not understand and possibly even misunderstands and which he feels has not been properly explained to him. Good communications between the patient and the health care team should be considered an important ingredient of good primary medical care. In the changing social climate of the 1970s, good communications are becoming increasingly important if not essential to the proper functioning of social, economic and political institutions. The methods and cost of communicating with a list of 3,000 patients of all ages, conditions and levels of intelligence presents numerous problems which are not easily resolved. However, good communications, as an important aspect of health education, are of such paramount importance that they deserve a higher priority in future than they have had in the past. It is perhaps relevant in this particular context to note that only 5 per cent of patients felt that the doctor did not explain and answer questions when they consulted him.

'Explanation before innovation' should be a maxim which is generally accepted as a guide not only by the professions providing the care but also by the family practitioner committees of the area health authorities. The patient cannot prescribe his own primary health care service but he is entitled to be informed and to have explained to him the nature and reasons for any changes which will affect him, most probably, at a time when he is not well and therefore likely to be apprehensive and perturbed. This may make it necessary to delay desirable innovations or not apply them to some patients in order to make certain that all who may be affected have had the fullest possible explanation.

More than 90 per cent of respondents of all ages and social classes were pleased that the doctor had an appointment system. This accords with the findings of other studies.[2] More than 25 per cent of all respondents did, however, give a positive reply to the question 'Have you ever had trouble getting an appointment to see your doctor?' This may have been related to the fact that about three out of five respondents had at some time wanted to see their doctor urgently, that is to say the same day. Appointment systems in general are well liked by patients but when the system appears unsatisfactory to them it can react unfavourably on patient-doctor relationships. Despite obvious problems with the appointment system which must have produced a great deal of patient/receptionist confrontation there was a general overall regard for the receptionists which is greatly to their credit. Widely looked upon as 'dragons at the gate' this particular group of receptionists found themselves well respected.

A good appointment system requires monitoring and the keeping of records which can show up any shortcomings. Both the receptionists and the patients should clearly understand the rules and procedure of the system and the doctor should be able to review at regular intervals the extent, if any, to which the system has not operated properly. The fact that 78 per cent of appointments are usually made by telephone illustrates the need for several telephone lines to the surgery. It was most surprising that about three out of five patients asked considered they had had reason to see the doctor urgently, i.e. that day. With this amount of immediate demand any appointment system in general practice that has not large numbers of vacant spaces available at the beginning of each working day is not going to satisfy patient demand. A sequel to this is that receptionists will attempt to apportion 'urgency' with all the problems that will follow from that. As a result of this particular statistic the appointment system in the Norton practice has been greatly amended with many more 'urgent' appointments available. It is interesting to note that of the patients who considered that they usually waited a long time on keeping an appointment (approximately one in six) over 50 per cent were annoyed or very annoyed. The days of gratitude for any sort of appointment system in place of the dreary wait in the crowded waiting room are now gone, and patients' expectations have been upgraded to expecting that an appoinment made at a specific time should be kept.

In addition to anxiety concerning less frequent contact with patients than normal in this particular practice there is also concern about the duration of the consultation in general practice as a whole. Five minutes is the much-quoted average and in this practice careful measurement showed it to be between five and six minutes. Nevertheless despite this speedy consultation over 90 per cent of those questioned felt that they were able to tell the doctor all they wanted to about their health, that the doctor always or often gave them sufficient time and didn't hurry them and that he nearly always explained things fully and answered all their questions. Very similar high satisfaction was expressed about the thoroughness of the examination and the carrying out of tests. It would seem that in the five-to six-minute consultation a great deal can be achieved.

In an earlier chapter considerable emphasis was placed on the way in which the personalised system of care minimised the doctor's workload. That 98 per cent of patients said they preferred a family doctor and approximately 80 per cent preferred to see him rather than the other doctors either at the surgery or at home suggests that one of the major workload-reducing systems is also popular with patients.

Although not especially related to workload it is of interest that over 25 per cent of the patients who needed a certificate of incapacity for work felt the doctor did not let them have one when they thought they needed one. Many employers look upon doctors as merely automatic legitimisers of absence – often for very trivial reasons – and this particular statistic certainly conflicts with that view.

Validity of the Findings

It is beyond reasonable doubt that the answers to the questions are representative of the sample selected for interview and it so happens, on account of the small divergences in the answers of various categories of patients, that they are representative of all the patients on the practice list. It is also very likely that the replies reflect quite genuinely the attitude of the respondents. Such a presumption can be no more than an inference from the pattern of replies and the comments reported by the interviewers. It is thus different from a statistical probability which is based on mathematical deductions.

The high esteem in which the British people hold the medical profession might discourage patients from criticising either their doctor or the conduct of his practice. There is also the possibility that respondents did not feel confident about the assurance they had received, that neither the doctor nor the other members of the health care team would see the replies which they made. If this confidence was lacking it might have discouraged respondents from replying truthfully. The answers to the questions do however show quite clearly that a substantial minority of patients were both satisfied with the overall service they received and yet quite critical of certain aspects of the service which they experienced. This seems to indicate candour and veracity. Furthermore, the replies show that when asked hypothetical questions, respondents have no difficulty in expressing definite views and do not resort to 'don't know' replies. The comments of respondents reported by interviewers are in a few cases more critical than the replies to the questions but this was sufficiently rare not to detract from the presumption that the replies in general reflect the genuine views of respondents.

The findings prove five out of the six hypotheses posed and give support to the other. They show up areas of patients' dissatisfaction and indicate a preference for the personal doctor system – approximately four out of five patients preferred to see their own doctor rather than another doctor in the group. The findings thus prove conclusively that the new style of health care described in Part I with its very low doctor workload *can* give a high level of satisfaction to some 90 per cent of all patients.

It is not however claimed or even suggested that the findings of this small survey of the patients of one practice are representative of all the people in Britain. They were inevitably much influenced by the personality and conduct of the doctor and the other members of the health care team.

The purpose of this survey was not to assess the level of patient satisfaction with general practitioner services in Britain but had the more specific object of assessing patient satisfaction with a system characterised by team care and a low doctor's workload. The monitoring of any social innovation presents inherent problems. Men who advocate changes are for that very reason not representative of their colleagues. They tend to be enthusiastic about the new ways, confident in the desirability of the change and for these reasons are often successful. It does not however necessarily follow that once the changes are generally adopted or enforced that the outcome will be equally successful. A new procedure or system worked by men who do not believe in it or by men less able to inspire confidence or by men inherently opposed to change may turn out rather differently from the results obtained when monitoring the innovation.

The conditions and attitude of mind which make the new style primary health care successful were summarised in an article in the *British Medical Journal*[3]:

> Given a desire to reduce and rationalise workload, given an attitude that patients should monitor their own short-term illnesses, given a delegation-orientated doctor and a team of readily available paramedical workers whose facilities are excellent, given a clinically confident and experienced general practitioner who does not devalue or minimise the training, experience and ability of the members of the team, given a known group of patients and even given an attitude which avoids hospital referral rather than seeks it, it would appear that even in a high morbidity and high mortality area, the workload of a general practitioner can become quite small . . .

and – we may now add – yet be compatible with a mere 2 per cent of patients expressing overall dissatisfaction with their primary health care.

The Role of Patient Satisfaction Surveys

These surveys are concerned with only one of the four dimensions of primary health care which are: (1) the workload of the team, (2) the patients' satisfaction with the service, (3) the quality of the service and (4) the extent to which it meets all needs and not merely all demands. Their limitations and usefulness must be assessed within this context.

In Part I, we have discussed the workload dimension and, on the limited data available, have made a prima facie case for the presumption that the Norton health care team provided a good quality service, in the sense that it compared favourably with published data whenever such comparisons could be made. The assessment of the quality of primary health care is generally acknowledged to be beset with difficulties and is widely and inconclusively debated in many countries.[4] Some of its distinctive features, in contrast to the evaluation of hospital care, have been well expressed by Ann Cartwright.[5]

> Methods of evaluating standards of care need to be developed which count as good care the *non*-investigation of symptoms which clear up quickly and spontaneously as well as the adequate investigation of conditions which need it. General practice should be assessed in terms of what it achieves and what it actually overlooks (not what it might be overlooking) rather than by its conformity to standards of care developed for hospital patients.

Systematic knowledge of achievement and shortcomings would in itself be an encouragement for the doctor to provide a high standard of care. Evaluation must be based on technical data and technical understanding; the patient as a layman is therefore not well placed to participate in this process. Evaluation of quality of service should be considered as an aspect of public accountability. The individual patient, as at present, is entitled to a conscientious and reasonable professional service, not to a service of a specific quality. This distinction is of crucial importance.

General practitioners are conscious of the danger of patients being over-demanding – an experience which all of them have encountered to a greater or lesser extent and from which they want to be protected. They tend to have less experience of the opposite danger – patients demanding too little and being too self-effacing. Such patients have a level of expectation which is so low that they suffer physical and mental disease and discomfort which, in the present state of medical knowledge and with the resources available, could be alleviated, arrested or remedied. The extent of such unmet needs is not known but there is some evidence that it is fairly widespread, especially among the elderly.[6,7]

There appears to be a sizeable proportion of people of all ages and a larger proportion of older people who consider the doctor to be an important and very busy man who cannot be expected to bother himself with their aches and pains. They, as well as others who do not share this view, suffer ill health with the same resignation or fortitude with which they face the common misfortunes of life, without realising that a visit to the surgery might greatly benefit them.

At present, public policy as well as medical opinion is ambivalent regarding unreported medical needs and the related issue of self-medication. Preventive screening for serious illnesses raises different issues but has the common feature of encouraging people to make demands on health services some of which are not even provided at present.

The shortage of medical manpower has been and is one of the major constraints on developments and policy changes in all three areas. The discussion of these complex and controversial issues which affect many different interests and which involves increased public expenditure is outside the scope of this study.

Two observations, however, are pertinent. The evolution of the new style of health care and especially its lower doctor's workload (which we have discussed in Part I) makes it possible to contemplate developments requiring medical manpower which would not otherwise have been possible. Decisions on the desirability of instituting programmes of screening particular population groups for specific diseases or of seeking out the unreported general medical needs of particular population groups, ought, in a democratic society, to be taken by politicians after appropriate discussion with doctors and administrators. The prevention, cure and retardation of fatal diseases will always be considered by medical and lay opinion alike as a matter of great importance but so is the relief of unnecessary and avoidable pain, suffering and discomfort. It seems to us rational as well as desirable that the cost of alternative policies should be assessed and the relevant issues debated before the political decisions are made.

We know of few systematic surveys of patient satisfaction with primary medical care services. When the Joint Working Party on General Medical Services 1973[8] wanted to acquaint themselves with the conditions currently prevailing in general practice and with the criticisms made against general medical services, they considered evidence from only two reports submitted to them: The Patients' Association[9] and Miss Proops of the *Daily Mirror*. Both of these were based on letters from self-selected correspondents and were rightly considered by the committee 'as necessarily biased'. The only other evidence they considered was a recent book[10] concerned with complaints about general practitioners to executive councils (now family practitioner committees).

Ann Cartwright's classical and original study *Patients and Their Doctors* was based on research undertaken in 1964 before 'the

Family Doctor's Charter' and well before the attachment of district nurses and health visitors to general practices. Bevan and Draper's study of patients' satisfaction with appointment systems was based on field work undertaken in 1963-5. Their findings, which were based on an interview survey undertaken by the British Market Research Bureau and a small postal survey of the patients of nine practices, are quite compatible with ours. A paper by Cunningham, Bevan and Floyd[11] which was based on a postal survey discusses the role of the practice nurse from the patient's point of view in a practice which serves part of a London borough. A comparison of its findings with ours cannot easily be made as the role of the nurse in that practice was not the same as that of the nurses in the practice which we surveyed.

The scarcity of published reports of patients' satisfaction with primary medical care may be due to some of the inherent difficulties in conducting such surveys. The joint working party remarked, 'General practitioners naturally tend to think in terms of the care of individuals, rather than of a more general responsibility to a community. As an independent contractor, the general practitioner does not expect detailed enquiry into the ways he provides services.' Another difficulty is the possibility that such surveys may undermine the relationship of trust which should exist between the patient and every member of the health care team. Such trust is not merely desirable but is a significant ingredient of certain aspects of therapy. It is therefore in the interest of both the doctor and the patient that surveys are conducted in such a way as to avoid the encouragement of dissatisfaction and mistrust among patients.

Social services nowadays are tending to become quite as client- and customer-orientated as commercial and fee-charging services have always been. In most developed countries, the trend towards patient-orientated health care is quite pronounced. This has manifested itself in Britain by the setting up of the Ombudsman and the Community Health Councils and the founding of the Patients' Association. Health care, whether purchased privately or provided as a communal service, does however differ markedly from other goods and services in some important respects related to its purpose and cost.

In the past, the object of commercial and other professional services was, to a large extent, the endeavour to maximise profits by satisfying the customers' or clients' demand. This was achieved by providing them with what they wanted at the right place, at the right time, at a price they were willing to pay and which compared not unfavourably with that charged by other suppliers. In recent decades, however, suppliers have become more and more aware that the object of the enterprise is often more effectively achieved by persuading people to buy what the supplier has to sell rather than by selling them what they would have wanted without this persuasion.

Health services have more complex objectives which occasionally conflict or appear to conflict with each other. Their purpose is not merely or even primarily to satisfy patients but to prevent, cure, alleviate and arrest disease, efficiently and expeditiously. Efficiently in this context means using the minimum resources and involving the least expense to achieve the set purpose. For patients of working age, a reduction in the length of illness which enables them to resume work earlier is another dimension of health care efficiency. Expeditiously means restoring the patient as quickly as possible to good health and/or to minimise the time during which he suffers unnecessary pain and discomfort.

Conflict thus arises when procedures which give much patient satisfaction – house calls by the doctor – are inefficient, or when efficient and effective methods – assessment visits by a nurse or routine ante-natal care by a midwife – leave some patients dissatisfied. A preventive screening programme for a particular disease might be popular with a large proportion of patients, but if the disease is rare and/or the probability of successful treatment even in the early stages of the disease is low, such a programme may be quite inefficient. The resources devoted to it would have been more effectively used in providing different types of services. Decisions of this kind are inherently difficult as they require a judgement on such issues as whether £10,000 spent on prolonging one life for a doubtful period is in some sense preferable to providing chiropody services for several hundred or even thousands of old people.

As patients are not able to judge the quality of the service they receive nor the quantity of the care they require it seems quite legitimate and proper to set out deliberately to persuade them to want what is in their own best interest and what can be provided efficiently. This is all the more important in primary health care where the patient's attitude towards the health care team may be a factor which affects his recovery. As an aside it is of interest to note that the purpose of health services, as we have defined them, could possibly be more efficiently attained by greater expenditure on health education aimed at discouraging people from smoking, overeating and excessive consumption of alcohol and encouraging them to take more exercise, than by the expenditure of the same sum on the building of district hospitals.

Satisfaction surveys in the primary health care field which ascertain the extent to which patients appreciate or object to specific aspects of the service can be seen to serve three purposes. First, if there is some dissatisfaction, to modify conduct or procedures where this is appropriate, by means compatible with the objects of the service. Second, where this is not appropriate, to review the possibility of persuading (educating) patients to want, or at least accept willingly, those aspects of the service with which they are dissatisfied. Third, if there is only minimal dissatisfaction, to establish that particular aspects of the service are acceptable to patients.

These surveys are especially useful when changes are contemplated or some time after they have been introduced.

There is scope and indeed need for local surveys, restricted to one or two practices, as well as for national surveys. Health care teams may wish to discover the reaction of their patients to innovations introduced by them, while the level of satisfaction with certain aspects of the service is a legitimate public concern. Surveys thus might lead to local or national changes in conduct and procedure where appropriate and to local or national endeavours to persuade (educate) people to accept changes.

The findings of such surveys should not be considered as an evaluation of the quality of primary health care but should be viewed as part of the trend to make the care more patient-orientated. They should provide useful indicators for the desirability of certain types of change but not conclusive arguments for changing all procedures and conduct which cause dissatisfaction. They should potentially contribute to reducing patient dissatisfaction though some degree of dissatisfaction with the service is of course unavoidable.

Notes

1. *The Times* (1975), 14 January 1975, p. 14.
2. Bevan, J.M. and Draper, G.J. (1967) *Appointment Systems in General Practice,* Oxford University Press, London.
3. Marsh, G.N. and McNay, R.A. (1974) *British Medical Journal,* 23 February 1974, pp.315-18.
4. Roemer, M.I. (1969) *The Organisation of Medical Care Under Social Security.* International Labour Office, Geneva (chapter 15).
5. Cartwright, Ann (1967) *Patients and Their Doctors.* Atherton Press, New York.
6. Yell, J. *et al, An Investigation Into the Social Conditions and Incidence of Treatable Disease Among Patients Aged 65 Years and Over in a 10,000 General Practice in Durham.* Durham Hospital Management Committee (mimeographed).
7. Williamson, J. *et al* (1964) Old People at Home; Their Unreported Needs. *Lancet,* 25 May 1964.
8. Department of Health and Social Security (1973) *General Medical Services, Report of Joint Working Party,* pp.2 and 3. HMSO, London.
9. *Patients and Their GPs* (1973) The Patients' Association (355 Gray's Inn Road London WC1).
10. Klein, R. (1973) *Complaints Against Doctors.* Charles Knight, London.
11. Cunningham, D.J. *et al* (1972) The role of the practice nurse from the patient's point of view. *Community Medicine,* 6 October 1972.

TABLES – PART II

Notes

In respect of each question asked the following information is given:

1. The percentage of the total population weighted by age group and sex of normal users and by aggregates of other categories of users (P).
2. The percentage of all respondents who gave the answers shown on the left-hand side, i.e. to Question 1 – YES, NO, DON'T KNOW (%).
3. The number of respondents who gave the answer shown on the left hand side (N).
4. The percentages of the five categories of users who gave the answers shown on the left-hand side. The categories are:

Normal	All users not belonging to any other category
CHB	Chronic housebound patients
Int-Care	Patients who received intensive care, i.e. saw the doctor twice a day on at least one occasion or three times in at least one week or five times in at least one month.
0-1	Users who did not see the doctor at all or only once during the year.
Nurse-first	Users who asked for a call by the doctor but were instead visited by a nurse.

5. The percentages of users in five age groups who gave the answers shown on the left-hand side.
6. The percentage of users in four social classes who gave the answers shown on the left-hand side. The social classes are:

I	Professional, managerial and skilled white-collar workers
II	Routine white-collar workers
III	Skilled manual workers
IV	Semi-skilled and unskilled manual workers

   The percentages for the five categories of users, the five age groups and the four social classes add up vertically for each column to 100 per cent.

   The numbers below the line add up horizontally for each of the three classifications to the appropriate number of respondents (N), while the corresponding percentages add up horizontally to 100 per cent.

   Any errors are due to rounding.

   Questions with an * beside them denote one CHB respondent whose social class could not be ascertained and who therefore could not be categorised.

   P.S. denotes a chi-square which is probably significant, i.e. < 0.05

   S denotes a chi-square which is significant, i.e. < 0.01

   H. S. denotes a chi-square which is highly significant, i.e. < 0.001

   In less than 5 per 100, 1 per 100, 1 per 1,000 times would the distributions shown happen by chance.

   Questions 46-50: The percentages given are the percentages of those who responded in the same category as in question 45.

   e.g. Normal users (column 1)

   187 responded in Q 45

   136 responded in Q 46

   So in Q 46 the percentage is found by calculating:

   $$\frac{136}{187} \times 100 = 72 \text{ per cent}$$

Table 34 Survey of Patient Satisfaction

KEY

			Category of User					Age Group					Social Class			
P	%	N	Nor-mal	CHB.	Int. Care	Nurse First	0-1 Users	16-19	20-34	35-49	50-64	65+	I	II	III	IV
	%	N	1	2	3	4	5	A	B	C	D	E	I	II	III	IV

Table 35

P		%	N	1	2	3	4	5	A	B	C	D	E	I	II	III	IV
	The Premises																
	Q.1 Have you been to the surgery during the past year?																
70%	Yes	88	276	94%		97%	100%	48%	85%	93%	88%	85%	84%	94%	90%	86%	82%
30%	No	12	39	6%		3%	0	52%	15%	7%	12%	15%	16%	6%	10%	14%	18%
0	Don't know	0	0	0		0	0	0	0	0	0	0	0	0	0	0	0
		100	315	187		35	43	50	34	88	80	52	61	65	74	95	81
				59%		11%	14%	16%	11%	28%	25%	17%	19%	21%	23%	30%	26%
								HS									
	Q.2 Do you have any difficulties getting to your doctor's surgery?																
7%	Yes	10	31	10%		11%	14%	6%	18%	8%	10%	4%	13%	6%	4%	13%	15%
91%	No	89	280	89%		86%	86%	92%	82%	92%	89%	90%	87%	94%	95%	84%	85%
2%	Sometimes	1	4	1%		3%	0	2%	0	0	1%	6%	0	0	1%	3%	0
		100	315	187		35	43	50	34	88	80	52	61	65	74	95	81
				59%		11%	14%	16%	11%	28%	25%	17%	19%	21%	23%	30%	26%
													PS				
	3-9. If Yes or Sometimes: what are the difficulties?																
Q.3	Difficult working hours?		2	1		0	1	0	1	0	1	0	0	0	0	1	1
Q.4	Small children at home?		1	0		0	0	1	0	0	1	0	0	0	0	0	1
Q.5	Long journey?		11	6		2	2	1	3	2	1	1	4	1	0	6	4
Q.6	Transportation problems?		17	9		3	4	1	2	4	4	3	4	1	4	7	5
Q.7	Parking problems?		None														
Q.8	Medical conditions?		5	2		1	1	1	0	1	1	2	1	0	0	4	1
Q.9	Other?		3	3		0	0	0	0	1	1	1	0	1	0	1	1

Table 36

P		%	N	1	2	3	4	5	A	B	C	D	E	I	II	III	IV
	Q.10 What are the practice premises like?																
52%	Excellent	60	189	63%		63%	67%	40%	29%	59%	66%	63%	67%	60%	66%	55%	60%
39%	Good	35	109	33%		34%	30%	46%	56%	35%	31%	33%	28%	38%	31%	35%	35%
9%	Don't know/average	5	17	4%		3%	2%	14%	15%	6%	3%	4%	5%	2%	3%	10%	5%
0	Poor	0	0	0		0	0	0	0	0	0	0	0	0	0	0	0
0	Very Poor	0	0	0		0	0	0	0	0	0	0	0	0	0	0	0
			315	187		35	43	50	34	88	80	52	61	65	74	95	81
		100		59%		11%	14%	16%	11%	28%	25%	17%	19%	21%	23%	30%	26%
								PS					PS				
	Q.11 Is there anything you would like to see changed about the waiting room?																
12%	Yes	12	38	13%		14%	7%	12%	18%	17%	14%	8%	3%	11%	20%	15%	2%
81%	No	86	270	87%		86%	93%	76%	76%	81%	85%	90%	95%	89%	74%	84%	95%
7%	Don't know	2	7	0		0	0	12%	6%	2%	1%	2%	2%	0	5%	1%	2%
			315	187		35	43	50	34	88	80	52	61	65	74	95	81
		100		59%		11%	14%	16%	11%	28%	25%	17%	19%	21%	23%	30%	26%
								HS									S
	Q.12 Is there a nurses' treatment room at the surgery?																
65%	Yes	75	235	77%		89%	79%	52%	47%	69%	84%	81%	80%	75%	77%	74%	73%
10%	No	7	22	6%		3%	7%	14%	18%	7%	5%	4%	7%	2%	11%	7%	7%
25%	Don't know	18	58	17%		9%	14%	34%	35%	24%	11%	15%	13%	23%	12%	19%	20%
			315	187		35	43	50	34	88	80	52	61	65	74	95	81
		100		59%		11%	14%	16%	11%	28%	25%	17%	19%	21%	23%	30%	26%
								S					S				

Table 37

P		%	N	1	2	3	4	5	A	B	C	D	E	I	II	III	IV
Q.13	If Yes: Have you had treatment in the nurses' treatment room?																
48%	Yes	54	129	56%		55%	59%	37%	59%	48%	48%	62%	63%	57%	55%	56%	49%
50%	No	45	108	44%		45%	41%	59%	41%	52%	51%	38%	37%	43%	43%	44%	51%
2%	Don't know	0	1	0		0	0	4%	0	0	1%	0	0	0	2%	0	0
			238	146		31	34	27	17	63	67	42	49	49	58	70	61
		100		61%		13%	14%	11%	7%	27%	28%	18%	21%	21%	24%	29%	26%
Q.14	If Yes: Is the treatment room equipped																
50%	Very well	53	69	52%		71%	50%	36%	9%	40%	47%	65%	77%	39%	62%	56%	52%
25%	Well	30	39	31%		18%	45%	18%	36%	40%	50%	12%	13%	46%	19%	28%	29%
25%	Don't know/averagely	17	22	17%		12%	5%	46%	55%	20%	3%	23%	10%	14%	19%	15%	19%
0	Poorly	0	0	0		0	0	0	0	0	0	0	0	0	0	0	0
0	Very poorly	0	0	0		0	0	0	0	0	0	0	0	0	0	0	0
			130	82		17	20	11	11	30	32	26	31	28	32	39	31
		100		63%		13%	15%	9%	8%	23%	25%	20%	24%	21%	25%	30%	24%

HS

Table 38

P		%	N	1	2	3	4	5	A	B	C	D	E	I	II	III	IV
	Part 2 – The Receptionists																
	Q.15 Have you ever spoken to a receptionist either at the surgery or on the telephone?																
89%*	Yes	90	306	96%	24%	100%	98%	86%	82%	99%	99%	94%	72%	97%	91%	89%	85%
11%	No	10	34	4%	76%	0	2%	14%	18%	1%	1%	6%	28%	3%	9%	11%	15%
0	Don't know	0	0	0	0	0	0	0	0	0	0	0	0	0	0	0	0
			340	187	25	35	43	50	34	88	81	55	82	69	78	103	89
		100		55%	7%	10%	13%	15%	10%	26%	24%	16%	24%	20%	23%	30%	26%
	If NO skip to Q.22																
								HS					HS				S
	Q.16 If Yes: In general do you find the receptionists who talk to you at the reception window or on the telephone are																
37%	Very pleasant	39	120	41%	17%	49%	36%	30%	14%	29%	40%	46%	59%	30%	44%	33%	51%
51%	Pleasant	48	147	45%	67%	40%	55%	58%	71%	52%	52%	38%	34%	58%	39%	53%	41%
10%	Don't know/Average	11	33	12%	0	11%	9%	9%	11%	16%	8%	12%	7%	10%	14%	11%	8%
1%	Unpleasant	1	4	2%	17%	0	0	0	4%	2%	0	2%	0	0	3%	2%	0
1%	Very unpleasant	1	2	1%	0	0	0	2%	0	1%	0	2%	0	2%	0	1%	0
			306	180	6	35	42	43	28	87	80	52	59	67	71	92	76
		100		59%	2%	11%	14%	14%	9%	28%	26%	17%	19%	22%	23%	30%	25%
													PS				
	Q.17 Are the receptionists																
0	Very unhelpful	1	2	1%	0	3%	0	0	0	0	0	4%	0	0	0	2%	0
3%	Unhelpful	2	7	1%	17%	3%	2%	5%	0	6%	0	4%	0	3%	3%	3%	0
6%	Don't know	5	15	6%	0	3%	2%	7%	0	6%	5%	6%	5%	6%	6%	3%	5%
56%	Helpful	56	171	56%	50%	51%	60%	58%	79%	54%	65%	48%	42%	52%	55%	62%	53%
35%	Very helpful	36	111	37%	33%	40%	36%	30%	21%	34%	30%	38%	53%	39%	37%	29%	42%
			306	180	6	35	42	43	28	87	80	52	59	67	71	92	76
		100		59%	2%	11%	14%	14%	9%	28%	26%	17%	19%	22%	23%	30%	25%
													S				

Table 39

P		%	N	1	2	3	4	5	A	B	C	D	E	I	II	III	IV
Q.18	Do the receptionists appear to be very concerned about you as																
9%	A patient	11	34	14%	0	14%	5%	5%	7%	10%	3%	22%	17%	7%	16%	10%	12%
55%	Concerned about you as a patient	56	171	57%	67%	54%	57%	52%	61%	56%	59%	51%	54%	51%	54%	58%	60%
15%	Don't know	12	36	10%	0	9%	17%	19%	11%	9%	11%	14%	15%	18%	7%	11%	12%
18%	Unconcerned about you as a patient	17	53	16%	17%	23%	17%	19%	21%	18%	25%	8%	12%	21%	19%	17%	13%
4%	Couldn't care less about you as a patient	4	11	3%	17%	0	5%	5%	0	6%	3%	6%	2%	3%	4%	4%	3%
		100	305	180 59%	6 2%	35 11%	42 14%	42 14%	28 9%	87 29%	80 26%	51 17%	59 19%	67 22%	70 23%	92 30%	76 25%
Q.19	Do the receptionists																
2%	Always rush you	2	7	1%	0	0	10%	2%	4%	1%	6%	0	0	3%	3%	2%	1%
5%	Usually rush you	6	19	6%	0	6%	10%	5%	11%	10%	8%	2%	0	10%	4%	9%	1%
18%	No opinion/indifferent	11	33	6%	33%	6%	14%	29%	7%	10%	10%	14%	12%	10%	17%	11%	5%
45%	Usually have time for you	46	140	49%	50%	49%	33%	43%	39%	58%	45%	33%	44%	54%	41%	41%	49%
30%	Always have time for you	35	106	38%	17%	40%	33%	21%	39%	21%	31%	51%	44%	22%	34%	37%	43%
		100	305	180 59%	6 2%	35 11%	42 14%	42 14%	28 9%	87 29%	80 26%	51 17%	59 19%	67 22%	70 23%	92 30%	76 25%
								S					S				

Table 40

P			%	N	1	2	3	4	5	A	B	C	D	E	I	II	III	IV
	Q.20	Do you feel they are																
79%		helping you get to the Doctor	76	233	80%	33%	74%	67%	79%	71%	71%	74%	82%	85%	72%	73%	73%	88%
10%		Neither helpful nor difficult	11	34	12%	33%	3%	14%	9%	11%	18%	11%	4%	7%	19%	13%	9%	5%
8%		Making it difficult for you to get to the doctor	10	29	7%	17%	17%	17%	7%	14%	10%	14%	10%	0	8%	11%	15%	3%
3%		Don't know	3	9	2%	17%	6%	2%	5%	4%	0	1%	4%	8%	1%	3%	3%	4%
				305	180	6	35	42	42	28	87	80	51	59	67	70	92	76
			100		59%	2%	11%	14%	14%	9%	29%	26%	17%	19%	22%	23%	30%	25%
														S				PS
	Q.21	Do you consider the receptionists																
68%		Give a good service	70	213	73%	50%	69%	67%	62%	46%	66%	69%	76%	83%	66%	66%	66%	82%
27%		Give an average service	26	80	24%	17%	29%	31%	31%	50%	33%	29%	18%	8%	30%	31%	28%	16%
2%		Give a poor service	1	4	1%	17%	0	0	2%	4%	1%	0	4%	0	0	1%	3%	0
3%		No opinion	3	8	2%	17%	3%	2%	5%	0	0	2%	2%	8%	4%	1%	2%	3%
				305	180	6	35	42	42	28	87	80	51	59	67	70	92	76
			100		59%	2%	11%	14%	14%	9%	29%	26%	17%	19%	22%	23%	30%	25%
														HS				
	Q.22	At the survery <u>do you</u> would you mind telling the receptionist why you want to see the doctor?																
18%		Yes	19	60	20%		14%	21%	16%	21%	24%	24%	11%	11%	23%	24%	18%	12%
71%		No	69	218	68%		74%	63%	74%	59%	60%	62%	83%	85%	68%	65%	67%	77%
9%		Sometimes	11	34	11%		9%	14%	8%	18%	16%	13%	6%	2%	9%	10%	14%	10%
1%		Don't know	1	3	0		3%	2%	2%	3%	0	1%	0	2%	0	1%	1%	1%
				315	187		35	43	50	34	88	80	52	61	65	74	95	81
			100		59%		11%	14%	16%	11%	28%	25%	17%	19%	21%	23%	30%	26%
														PS				

Table 41

do you

Q.23 At the surgery would you mind telling a qualified nurse why you want to see the doctor?

P			%	N	1	2	3	4	5	A	B	C	D	E	I	II	III	IV
6%		Yes	5	16	6%		3%	2%	6%	0	6%	5%	8%	5%	3%	5%	5%	6%
93%		No	91	288	91%		91%	88%	94%	97%	91%	90%	88%	93%	94%	91%	92%	90%
1%		Sometimes	3	9	2%		6%	9%	0	3%	2%	5%	4%	0	2%	3%	3%	4%
0		Don't know	1	2	1%		0	0	0	0	1%	0	0	2%	2%	1%	0	0
				315	187		35	43	50	34	88	80	52	61	65	74	95	81
			100		59%		11%	14%	16%	11%	28%	25%	17%	19%	21%	23%	30%	26%

do you

Q.24 On the telephone would you mind telling the receptionist the reason why you want a home visit by the doctor?

P			%	N	1	2	3	4	5	A	B	C	D	E	I	II	III	IV
14%	*	Yes	11	37	10%	5%	0	19%	20%	23%	11%	9%	11%	8%	14%	7%	16%	7%
81%		No	81	271	85%	47%	100%	67%	78%	71%	81%	85%	89%	76%	80%	92%	73%	82%
3%		Sometimes	5	16	4%	5%	0	14%	2%	6%	8%	6%	0	3%	6%	1%	6%	6%
1%		Don't know	3	10	1%	42	0	0	0	0	0	0	0	13%	0	0	5%	5%
				344	187	19	35	43	50	34	88	81	55	76	69	77	102	85
			100		56%	6%	10%	13%	15%	10%	26%	24%	17%	23%	21%	23%	31%	25%
									HS					HS				HS

do you

Q.25 On the telephone would you mind telling a qualified nurse the reason why you want a home visit by the doctor?

P			%	N	1	2	3	4	5	A	B	C	D	E	I	II	III	IV
5%	*	Yes	4	12	4%	0	0	5%	6%	9%	6%	1%	2%	3%	4%	1%	6%	2%
94%		No	93	311	94%	63%	100%	95%	94%	91%	93%	98%	98%	85%	94%	99%	88%	94%
0		Sometimes	1	2	1%	0	0	0	0	0	1%	1%	0	0	1%	0	1%	0
1%		Don't know	3	9	1%	37%	0	0	0	0	0	0	0	12%	0	0	5%	4%
				334	187	19	35	43	50	34	88	81	55	76	69	77	102	85
			100		56%	6%	10%	13%	15%	10%	26%	24%	17%	23%	21%	23%	31%	25%
									HS					HS				HS

Table 42		%	N	1	2	3	4	5	A	B	C	D	E	I	II	III	IV
P																	
Q.26 Would you mind the receptionist giving you a message from the doctor (e.g. about the result of tests)?																	
25% *	Yes	21	70	18%	14%	23%	26%	30%	35%	16%	23%	27%	13%	13%	25%	25%	18%
65%	No	69	234	76%	43%	69%	70%	58%	65%	75%	74%	65%	64%	77%	68%	64%	74%
8%	Sometimes	6	19	5%	0	6%	5%	12%	0	9%	3%	4%	9%	9%	6%	5%	3%
2%	Don't know	4	13	2%	43%	3%	0	0	0	0	0	4%	14%	1%	1%	6%	5%
			336	187	21	35	43	50	34	88	81	55	78	69	77	102	87
		100		56%	6%	10%	13%	15%	10%	26%	24%	16%	23%	21%	23%	30%	26%
								HS					HS				HS
Do you Q.27 Would you mind the receptionist enquiring from the doctor about some treatment for you?																	
21% *	Yes	23	77	23%	25%	20%	33%	18%	35%	23%	25%	24%	16%	29%	29%	22%	15%
67%	No	66	221	68%	40%	74%	60%	68%	62%	70%	62%	67%	66%	59%	60%	66%	78%
11%	Sometimes	7	25	7%	0	3%	7%	14%	3%	6%	14%	7%	5%	10%	10%	8%	2%
2%	Don't know	4	12	2%	35%	3%	0	0	0	1%	0	2%	13%	1%	1%	5%	5%
			335	187	20	35	43	50	34	88	81	55	77	69	77	102	86
		100		56%	6%	10%	13%	15%	10%	26%	24%	16%	23%	21%	23%	30%	26%
								HS					HS				HS
Do you Q.28 Would you mind getting advice about your health from a receptionist?																	
73% *	Yes	72	241	71%	55%	86%	74%	72%	71%	73%	83%	73%	60%	74%	77%	72%	66%
22%	No	22	73	23%	20%	14%	23%	24%	23%	19%	16%	20%	31%	20%	19%	20%	28%
3%	Sometimes	4	13	6%	0	0	2%	2%	6%	7%	1%	5%	1%	3%	4%	5%	4%
2%	Don't know	2	8	1%	25%	0	0	2%	0	1%	0	2%	8%	3%	0	4%	2%
			335	187	20	35	43	50	34	88	81	55	77	69	77	102	86
		100		56%	6%	10%	13%	15%	10%	26%	24%	16%	23%	21%	23%	30%	26%
								HS					PS				

Table 43

P		%	N	1	2	3	4	5	A	B	C	D	E	I	II	III	IV
	Q.29 Have you ever received advice about your health from a qualified nurse?																
18%*	Yes	29	99	21%	76%	37%	53%	10%	15%	36%	27%	18%	37%	29%	27%	31%	28%
82%	No	71	240	79%	20%	63%	47%	90%	85%	64%	73%	82%	62%	71%	73%	69%	71%
0	Sometimes	0	1	0	4%	0	0	0	0	0	0	0	4%	0	0	0	1%
0	Don't know	0	0	0	0	0	0	0	0	0	0	0	0	0	0	0	0
			340	187	25	35	43	50	34	88	81	55	82	69	78	103	89
		100		55%	7%	10%	13%	15%	10%	26%	24%	16%	24%	20%	23%	30%	26%
								HS									
	Q.30 Did you / Would you mind?																
11%*	Yes	10	33	11%	4%	3%	12%	10%	6%	5%	21%	14%	2%	9%	13%	9%	9%
80%	No	83	282	83%	96%	91%	79%	78%	91%	84%	70%	82%	94%	79%	79%	86%	86%
9%	Sometimes	6	21	5%	0	6%	9%	12%	0	11%	8%	4%	4%	10%	7%	5%	5%
0	Don't know	1	2	1%	0	0	0	0	3%	0	1%	0	0	2%	1%	0	0
			338	187	24	34	43	50	34	88	80	55	81	68	77	103	89
		100		55%	7%	10%	13%	15%	10%	26%	24%	16%	24%	20%	23%	30%	26%
													HS				

Table 44

P		%	N	1	2	3	4	5	A	B	C	D	E	I	II	III	IV
	Part 3 – The Appointment System																
	Q.31 When you want to see the doctor how do you usually make your appointment?																
49%*	Use your own telephone	44	150	46%	24%	37%	44%	52%	38%	53%	56%	44%	26%	77%	56%	33%	21%
29%	Use a public telephone	28	94	28%	0	34%	35%	30%	32%	31%	28%	40%	13%	9%	20%	36%	39%
13%	Go to the surgery	15	50	18%	0	20%	9%	10%	15%	13%	15%	11%	20%	9%	12%	17%	19%
6%	Have someone else phone	10	33	6%	52%	9%	9%	4%	9%	2%	1%	4%	30%	4%	5%	11%	16%
1%	Have someone else go to the surgery	2	6	2%	4%	0	2%	0	3%	1%	0	2%	4%	1%	3%	2%	1%
2%	Haven't made appt./not appl.	1	4	0	8%	0	0	4%	3%	0	0	0	4%	0	3%	0	2%
0	Tell nurse or home help	1	3	0	12%	0	0	0	0	0	0	0	4%	0	1%	1%	1%
			340	187	25	35	43	50	34	88	81	55	82	69	78	103	89
		100		55%	7%	10%	13%	15%	10%	26%	24%	16%	24%	20%	23%	30%	26%
								HS					HS				HS
	Q.32 Are you pleased your doctor has an appointment system?																
87%	Yes	91	286	92%		94%	91%	82%	82%	90%	92%	94%	92%	91%	95%	90%	89%
7%	No	7	21	6%		6%	9%	8%	9%	9%	5%	4%	7%	8%	4%	7%	7%
6%	Don't know/Don't care	2	8	2%		0	0	10%	9%	1%	3%	2%	2%	1%	1%	3%	4%
			315	187		35	43	50	34	88	80	52	61	65	74	95	81
		100		59%		11%	14%	16%	11%	28%	25%	17%	19%	21%	23%	30%	26%
								PS									
	Q.33 Have you ever had trouble getting an appointment to see your doctor?																
24%	Yes	28	87	27%		31%	35%	22%	29%	40%	31%	19%	11%	25%	34%	32%	20%
72%	No	71	224	73%		69%	63%	72%	65%	60%	69%	79%	87%	75%	65%	66%	79%
3%	Don't know	1	4	0		0	2%	6%	6%	0	0	2%	2%	0	1%	2%	1%
			315	187		35	43	50	34	88	80	52	61	65	74	95	81
		100		59%		11%	14%	16%	11%	28%	25%	17%	19%	21%	23%	30%	26%
								PS					S				

Table 45

P		%	N	1	2	3	4	5	A	B	C	D	E	I	II	III	IV
	Q.34 Have you ever wanted to see your doctor urgently (i.e. that day)?																
47%*	Yes	59	201	56%	72%	83%	74%	34%	38%	65%	64%	60%	56%	56%	62%	54%	65%
53%	No	41	139	44%	28%	17%	26%	66%	62%	35%	36%	40%	44%	44%	38%	46%	35%
0	Don't know	0	0	0	0	0	0	0	0	0	0	0	0	0	0	0	0
			340	187	25	35	43	50	34	88	81	55	82	69	78	103	89
		100		55%	7%	10%	13%	15%	10%	26%	24%	16%	24%	20%	23%	30%	26%
	If no or don't know skip to Q.39							HS									
	Q.35 If Yes: Could you see your own doctor?																
64%	Yes	60	120	56%	56%	69%	59%	71%	38%	47%	71%	70%	61%	59%	58%	57%	64%
28%	No	27	54	31%	22%	21%	22%	19%	54%	26%	25%	18%	28%	18%	35%	29%	24%
8%	Sometimes/Don't know	13	27	13%	22%	10%	19%	0	8%	26%	4%	12%	11%	23%	6%	14%	12%
			201	105	18	29	32	17	13	57	52	33	46	39	48	56	58
		100		52%	9%	14%	16%	9%	7%	28%	26%	16%	23%	19%	24%	28%	29%
	If yes skip to Q.39												PS				
	Q.36 If no: were you seen by another doctor?																
69%	Yes	81	44	84%	75%	100%	86%	40%	57%	100%	77%	83%	77%	86%	88%	75%	79%
31%	No	19	10	16%	25%	0	14%	60%	43%	0	23%	17%	23%	14%	12%	25%	21%
			54	32	4	6	7	5	7	15	13	6	13	7	17	16	14
		100		59%	7%	11%	13%	9%	13%	28%	24%	11%	24%	13%	31%	30%	26%
	If Yes skip to Q.39																
	Q.37 Were you seen by a nurse?																
27%	Yes	17	2	0	50%		0	33%	0	0	0	0	67%	0	50%	0	25%
73%	No	83	10	100%	50%		100%	67%	100%	100%	100%	100%	33%	100%	50%	100%	75%
0	Dont know	0	0	0	0		0	0	0	0	0	0	0	0	0	0	0
			12	5	2		2	3	3	1	3	2	3	1	2	5	4
		100		42%	17%		17%	25%	25%	8%	25%	17%	25%	8%	17%	42%	33%

Table 46

P		%	N	1	2	3	4	5	A	B	C	D	E	I	II	III	IV
Q.38 If you were not seen by a doctor do you feel your health suffered?																	
14%	Yes	40	4	80%	0		0	0	67%		0	100%	33%	0	50%	75%	0
87%	No	60	6	20%	100%		100%	100%	33%		100%	0	67%	100%	50%	25%	100%
0	Don't know	0	0	0	0		0	0	0		0	0	0	0	0	0	0
			10	5	1		1	3	3		3	1	3	1	2	4	3
		100		50%	10%		10%	30%	30%		30%	10%	30%	10%	20%	40%	30%
Q.39 When you had an urgent problem did you mind explaining the urgency to the receptionist? (If you … would you)																	
13%*	Yes	13	44	13%	5%	14%	16%	12%	18%	11%	14%	26%	4%	13%	11%	16%	13%
82%	No	81	270	82%	70%	83%	77%	82%	82%	84%	80%	74%	82%	81%	83%	82%	77%
4%	Sometimes	4	13	3%	0	3%	7%	6%	0	5%	6%	0	5%	6%	5%	0	6%
1%	Don't know	2	7	1%	25%	0	0	0	0	0	0	0	9%	0	1%	2%	5%
			334	186	20	35	43	50	34	88	81	54	77	69	76	102	86
		100		51%	6%	10%	13%	15%	10%	26%	24%	16%	23%	21%	23%	30%	26%
								HS					HS				
Q.40 On keeping an appointment do you find you usually have to wait a long time?																	
17%	Yes	24	74	25%		31%	26%	12%	41%	33%	25%	12%	8%	29%	29%	22%	16%
78%	No	74	232	74%		69%	72%	80%	56%	64%	75%	84%	89%	69%	70%	76%	79%
5%	Don't know	2	8	2%		0	2%	8%	3%	3%	0	4%	3%	2%	1%	2%	5%
			314	186		35	43	50	34	88	80	51	61	65	73	95	81
		100		59%		11%	14%	16%	11%	28%	26%	16%	19%	21%	23%	30%	26%
													S				

Table 47

P		%	N	1	2	3	4	5	A	B	C	D	E	1	2	3	4
	Q.41 If Yes: are you																
14%	Very annoyed	14	10	11%		18%	18%	17%	14%	7%	20%	17%	20%	0	24%	10%	23%
46%	Annoyed	37	27	33%		27%	46%	67%	29%	38%	50%	17%	20%	42%	38%	33%	31%
14%	Don't know/Indifferent	20	15	17%		46%	18%	0	14%	31%	5%	33%	20%	21%	19%	19%	23%
20%	Happy to Wait	28	21	39%		9%	18%	0	43%	24%	25%	17%	40%	37%	19%	38%	15%
6%	Very happy to wait	1	1	0		0	0	17%	0	0	0	17%	0	0	0	0	8%
			74	46		11	11	6	14	29	20	6	5	19	21	21	13
		100		62%		15%	15%	8%	19%	39%	27%	8%	7%	26%	28%	28%	18%
								PS									

Table 48

P		%	N	1	2	3	4	5	A	B	C	D	E	I	II	III	IV
	Part 4 – The Personal Doctor System																
	Q.42 Are you aware that each doctor in the practice has his own list of patients?																
94%*	Yes	92	313	92%	80%	94%	93%	96%	85%	96%	99%	89%	87%	99%	94%	91%	86%
4%	No	4	15	5%	8%	6%	0	2%	9%	3%	1%	4%	7%	0	4%	7%	6%
2%	Don't know	4	12	3%	12%	0	7%	2%	6%	1%	0	7%	6%	1%	3%	2%	8%
			340	187	25	35	43	50	34	88	81	55	82	69	78	103	89
		100		55%	7%	10%	13%	15%	10%	26%	24%	16%	24%	20%	23%	30%	26%
	Q.43 How did you come to be registered with your doctor?																
9% *	Registered by previous doctor	13	43	13%	16%	9%	19%	6%	6%	9%	16%	4%	22%	14%	17%	13%	8%
8%	Reg. by relatives	12	40	14%	4%	23%	7%	2%	18%	19%	10%	2%	10%	14%	12%	12%	10%
10%	Reg. by friends, neighbours workmates	11	36	13%	8%	0	14%	8%	6%	17%	10%	15%	4%	19%	12%	11%	3%
10%	Alloc. By Receptionist	11	39	13%	4%	14%	12%	8%	9%	18%	10%	9%	8%	10%	15%	7%	15%
53%	Always in practice	44	151	38%	60%	37%	44%	66%	53%	31%	42%	54%	51%	33%	36%	47%	57%
10%	Other	9	31	9%	8%	17%	5%	10%	9%	6%	12%	16%	5%	9%	9%	12%	7%
			340	187	25	35	43	50	34	88	81	55	82	69	78	103	89
		100		55%	7%	10%	13%	15%	10%	26%	24%	16%	24%	20%	23%	30%	26%
								PS					HS				
	Q.44 In the surgery do you prefer to see your own doctor?																
35%	Strongly	39	123	36%		49%	53%	32%	15%	39%	37%	46%	49%	35%	39%	45%	35%
44%	Preferably	43	135	45%		43%	33%	42%	50%	43%	54%	31%	34%	48%	39%	35%	52%
0	It depends	0	1	0		0	2%	0	0	1%	0	0	0	2%	0	0	0
18%	Don't mind	16	50	17%		9%	12%	22%	35%	16%	8%	17%	15%	14%	22%	18%	10%
3%	Couldn't care less	2	6	2%		0	0	4%	0	1%	1%	6%	2%	2%	0	2%	4%
			315	187		35	43	50	34	88	80	52	61	65	74	95	81
		100		59%		11%	14%	16%	11%	28%	25%	17%	19%	21%	23%	30%	26%
													S				

Table 49

P		%	N	1	2	3	4	5	A	B	C	D	E	I	II	III	IV
	Q.45 At home do you prefer to see your own doctor (i.e. your family)																
32%*	Strongly	36	123	36%	28%	46%	44%	28%	24%	32%	35%	40%	45%	25%	35%	51%	29%
41%	Preferably	42	142	40%	52%	49%	40%	40%	35%	42%	52%	36%	38%	52%	40%	27%	52%
1%	It depends	1	2	1%	0	0	0	2%	0	0	1%	2%	0	1%	0	1%	0
22%	Don't mind	19	66	21%	20%	6%	16%	26%	38%	25%	11%	16%	16%	20%	26%	18%	16%
3%	Couldn't care less	2	7	3%	0	0	0	4%	3%	1%	1%	6%	1%	1%	0	3%	3%
			340	187	25	35	43	50	34	88	81	55	82	69	78	103	89
		100		55%	7%	10%	13%	15%	10%	26%	24%	16%	24%	20%	23%	30%	26%

(If responses to 44 and 45 are 4 or 5, skip to Q.52)

PS

For the following question the respondent may answer yes as many times as are applicable

46-50: If preferable: why is it that you prefer your own doctor? Is it that

	N	1	2	3	4	5	A	B	C	D	E	I	II	III	IV
Q.46 * He knows and understands you	251	136	17	29	37	32	18	66	67	41	59	50	56	77	67
		72%	68%	83%	86%	64%	53%	75%	83%	75%	72%	72%	72%	75%	75%
Q.47 *You know and understand him	204	111	14	25	28	26	15	41	61	36	51	44	44	62	53
		59%	56%	71%	65%	52%	44%	47%	75%	65%	62%	64%	56%	60%	60%
Q.48 * You trust him	197	106	17	25	24	25	15	45	51	29	57	42	41	59	54
		57%	68%	71%	56%	50%	44%	51%	63%	53%	70%	61%	53%	57%	61%
Q.49 He is better than the other doctors	57	37	2	8	6	4	9	15	10	13	10	13	9	24	11
		20%	8%	23%	14%	8%	26%	17%	12%	24%	12%	19%	12%	23%	12%
Q.50 Other reasons	33	19	3	5	2	4	1	10	8	6	8	5	3	9	16
		10%	12%	14%	5%	8%	• 3%	11%	10%	11%	10%	7%	4%	9%	18%

Table 50

P		%	N	1	2	3	4	5	A	B	C	D	E	I	II	III	IV
Q.51 Have you ever wished you could consult another doctor in the practice?																	
9% *	Yes	7	20	6%	4%	6%	11%	10%	0	11%	7%	9%	4%	7%	14%	6%	3%
91	No	93	264	94%	96%	94%	89%	90%	100%	89%	93%	91%	96%	93%	86%	94%	97%
0	Don't know	0	0	0	0	0	0	0	0	0	0	0	0	0	0	0	0
			284	150	25	33	37	39	21	73	74	44	72	58	64	83	78
		100		53%	9%	12%	13%	14%	7%	26%	26%	16%	25%	20%	22%	29%	28%
Q.52 (For female patients) Would you like to be able to consult a lady doctor?																	
64%	Yes	11	24	10%	9%	5%	10%	21%	12%	9%	8%	16%	13%	6%	19%	8%	10%
28%	No	79	174	78%	77%	90%	80%	75%	53%	87%	81%	78%	76%	85%	72%	80%	79%
7%	Sometimes	7	15	10%	5%	5%	2%	4%	29%	3%	8%	6%	4%	6%	7%	7%	7%
1%	Don't know	3	7	2%	9%	0	8%	0	6%	1%	2%	0	7%	2%	2%	5%	4%
			220	115	22	19	40	24	17	68	48	32	55	48	54	61	57
		100		52%	10%	9%	18%	11%	8%	31%	22%	14%	25%	22%	24%	28%	26%
													PS				
Q.53 As far as the treatment you receive from your doctor, in general, would you say you were																	
47%*	Very satisfied	49	166	51%	32%	57%	49%	44%	26%	49%	47%	58%	54%	49%	50%	48%	48%
41%	Satisfied	43	148	43%	60%	43%	39%	40%	65%	42%	44%	33%	43%	48%	41%	41%	46
10%	Don't know/mixed feelings	6	20	5%	0	0	7%	14%	6%	9%	6%	5%	2%	3%	9%	8%	3%
1%	Dissatisfied	2	5	0	8%	0	5%	2%	3%	0	3%	2%	1%	0	0	3%	2%
0	Very dissatisfied	0	1	1%	0	0	0	0	0	0	0	2%	0	0	0	1%	0
			340	187	25	35	43	50	34	88	81	55	82	69	78	103	89
		100		55%	7%	10%	13%	15%	10%	26%	24%	16%	24%	20%	23%	30%	26%
								PS									

Table 51

P		%	N	1	2	3	4	5	A	B	C	D	E	I	II	III	IV
Q.54 Do you feel that you are able to tell your doctor all you want to about your health?																	
89%*	Yes	91	308	90%	96%	94%	91%	88%	91%	90%	89%	85%	96%	88%	87%	88%	98%
6%	No	6	21	6%	0	6%	9%	6%	9%	7%	7%	7%	2%	7%	9%	8%	1%
3%	Sometimes	2	8	3%	4%	0	0	2%	0	2%	4%	4%	1%	3%	4%	3%	0
2%	Don't know	1	3	1%	0	0	0	4%	0	1%	0	4%	0	1%	0	1%	1%
			340	187	25	35	43	50	34	88	81	55	82	69	78	103	89
		100		55%	7%	10%	13%	15%	10%	26%	24%	16%	24%	20%	23%	30%	26%
Q.55 Do you feel you are able to consult him about more than one condition at any one attendance?																	
82%*	Yes	84	285	81%	96%	91%	86%	80%	79%	81%	84%	80%	92%	78%	78%	87%	89%
10%	No	13	43	18%	0	9%	9%	4%	12%	17%	15%	14%	5%	19%	21%	8%	7%
2%	Sometimes	1	5	1%	0	0	5%	4%	3%	1%	0	2%	2%	3%	0	2%	1%
6%	Don't know	2	7	0	4%	0	0	12%	6%	1%	1%	4%	1%	0	1%	3%	3%
			340	187	25	35	43	50	34	88	81	55	82	69	78	103	89
		100		55%	7%	10%	13%	15%	10%	26%	24%	16%	24%	20%	23%	30%	26%
	<u>Do you</u>							HS									
Q.56 Would you feel that you are able to talk to your doctor about problems or difficulties which are not medical?																	
64%	Yes	69	236	72%	72%	77%	67%	56%	65%	68%	74%	74%	65%	65%	69%	69%	73%
27%*	No	21	71	20%	12%	20%	16%	34%	26%	25%	17%	20%	18%	28%	23%	20%	15%
1%	Sometimes	2	5	1%	4%	0	5%	2%	0	1%	1%	2%	2%	1%	1%	3%	0
8%	Don't know	8	28	3%	12%	3%	12%	8%	9%	6%	7%	4%	15%	6%	6%	8%	12%
			340	187	25	35	43	50	34	88	81	55	82	69	78	103	89
		100		55%	7%	10%	13%	15%	10%	26%	24%	16%	24%	20%	23%	30%	26%

Table 52

P		%	N	1	2	3	4	5	A	B	C	D	E	I	II	III	IV
Q.57	Do you feel your doctor gives you sufficient time and doesn't hurry you?																
72% *	Always	76	259	80%	80%	80%	70%	64%	71%	68%	77%	78%	85%	72%	69%	76%	85%
11%	Often	14	48	13%	8%	20%	21%	10%	26%	22%	14%	2%	10%	22%	15%	14%	8%
8%	Don't know	4	12	2%	8%	0	0	14%	3%	3%	1%	5%	5%	3%	4%	2%	6%
9%	Seldom	5	18	5%	4%	0	5%	12%	0	6%	7%	13%	0	3%	10%	7%	1%
0	Never	1	3	1%	0	0	5%	0	0	1%	1%	2%	0	0	1%	2%	0
			340	187	25	35	43	50	34	88	81	55	82	69	78	103	89
		100		55%	7%	10%	13%	15%	10%	26%	24%	16%	24%	20%	23%	30%	26%
								HS					S				
Q.58	Do you feel your doctor gives you a thorough examination when necessary?																
78% *	Yes	85	289	89%	92%	89%	83%	68%	79%	86%	83%	89%	87%	84%	90%	85%	82%
7%	No	6	19	4%	4%	3%	12%	10%	3%	6%	10%	4%	4%	7%	4%	8%	3%
4%	Sometimes	3	10	2%	4%	9%	2%	4%	3%	5%	4%	0	2%	4%	3%	1%	5%
11%	Don't know	6	21	6%	0	0	2%	18%	15%	3%	4%	7%	7%	4%	4%	6%	10%
			339	187	25	35	42	50	34	87	81	55	82	69	78	102	89
		100		55%	7%	10%	12%	15%	10%	26%	24%	16%	24%	20%	23%	30%	26%
								S									
Q.59	Do you think your doctor undertakes all necessary tests?																
78% *	Yes	77	263	80%	84%	94%	72%	56%	62%	75%	75%	82%	85%	75%	83%	74%	78%
9%	No	8	27	6%	4%	6%	14%	12%	6%	9%	16%	5%	1%	13%	6%	9%	4%
16%	Not applicable	11	37	11%	12%	0	2%	24%	29%	9%	9%	9%	9%	9%	9%	12%	14%
6%	Don't know	4	13	2%	0	0	12%	8%	3%	7%	0	4%	5%	3%	1%	6%	4%
			340	187	25	35	43	50	34	88	81	55	82	69	78	103	89
		100		55%	7%	10%	13%	15%	10%	26%	24%	16%	24%	20%	23%	30%	26%
								HS					S				

Table 53

P		%	N	1	2	3	4	5	A	B	C	D	E	I	II	III	IV
	Q.60 Do you think your doctor refers you to hospital																
1%*	Too often	1	4	1%	0	0	2%	2%	0	2%	1%	2%	0	1%	4%	0	0
46%	Just right	53	178	48%	76%	69%	63%	38%	41%	49%	60%	60%	49%	59%	47%	50%	54%
2%	Not enough	3	10	3%	4%	6%	2%	0	6%	3%	3%	4%	1%	3%	1%	4%	3%
48%	Not applicable	41	140	45%	20%	26%	33%	56%	53%	43%	32%	34%	48%	33%	46%	44%	40%
3%	Don't know	2	7	3%	0	0	0	4%	0	2%	4%	0	2%	3%	1%	2%	2%
			339	186	25	35	43	50	34	88	80	55	82	69	78	102	89
		100		55%	7%	10%	13%	15%	10%	26%	24%	16%	24%	20%	23%	30%	26%
	Q.61 Do you feel your doctor lets you have a certificate when you think you need one?																
30% *	Yes	26	87	27%	0	37%	16%	32%	44%	28%	24%	38%	9%	32%	22%	19%	33%
13%	No	11	38	12%	0	17%	9%	12%	6%	11%	20%	14%	2%	7%	15%	14%	8%
2%	Sometimes	2	7	3%	0	3%	0	2%	3%	2%	3%	4%	0	3%	1%	3%	1%
51%	Not applicable	60	202	57%	100	43%	74%	48%	44%	56%	51%	44%	89%	57%	62%	64%	55%
4%	Don't know	1	5	1%	0	0	0	6%	3%	2%	3%	0	0	1%	0	1%	3%
			339	186	25	35	43	50	34	88	80	55	82	69	78	102	89
		100		55%	7%	10%	13%	15%	10%	26%	24%	16%	24%	20%	23%	30%	26%
								S			HS						
	Q.62 Do you feel your doctor prescribes medicines																
1% *	Too readily	2	6	3%	0	0	2%	0	6%	2%	1%	2%	0	1%	0	3%	2%
81%	Just right	88	297	90%	100%	97%	79%	72%	79%	88%	90%	89%	88%	94%	87%	83%	90%
1%	Not often enough	1	5	1%	0	0	7%	0	6%	0	3%	0	1%	0	3%	3%	0%
14%	Not applicable	7	24	4%	0	3%	9%	24%	9%	4%	6%	7%	10%	6%	10%	7%	6%
3%	Don't know	2	7	2%	0	0	2%	4%	0	6%	0	2%	1%	1%	0	4%	2%
			339	186	25	35	43	50	34	88	80	55	82	69	78	102	89
		100		55%	7%	10%	13%	15%	10%	26%	24%	16%	24%	20%	23%	30	26%
								HS									

Table 54

P		%	N	1	2	3	4	5	A	B	C	D	E	I	II	III	IV
Q.63 Do you feel your doctor, explains things to you fully and answers all your questions?																	
80% *	Yes	85	289	88%	88%	89%	84%	74%	82%	85%	83%	85%	89%	85%	83%	88%	83%
6%	No	5	18	4%	8%	3%	9%	8%	6%	6%	6%	9%	1%	3%	9%	4%	6%
10%	Sometimes	7	24	6%	4%	9%	7%	12%	6%	8%	11%	2%	6%	9%	8%	7%	6%
4%	Don't know	2	8	3%	0	0	0	6%	6%	1%	0	4%	4%	3%	0	1%	6%
			339	186	25	35	43	50	34	88	80	55	82	69	78	102	89
		100		55	7%	10%	13%	15%	10%	26%	24%	16%	24%	20%	23%	30%	26%
Q.64 In your experience would you say that your doctor																	
29%*	Is very concerned about your problems	31	104	30%	28%	43%	33%	24%	15%	33%	27%	38%	33%	23%	28%	35%	33%
61%	Is concerned about your problems	61	207	64%	52%	51%	58%	62%	79%	57%	69%	53%	55%	74%	63%	54%	57%
6%	Don't know	5	17	3%	16%	3%	7%	8%	6%	3%	1%	4%	11%	0	4%	7%	8%
3%	Is unconcerned about your problems	3	10	3%	4%	3%	2%	4%	0	6%	3%	5%	0	1%	5%	4%	1%
1%	Couldn't care less	1	2	1%	0	0	0	2%	0	1%	0	0	1%	1%	0	0	1%
			340	187	25	35	43	50	34	88	81	55	82	69	78	103	89
		100		55%	7%	10%	13%	15%	10%	26%	24%	16%	24%	20%	23%	30%	26%
													PS				
Q.65 Would you say that your relationship with your doctor is a businesslike one only, or do you feel it is friendly too?																	
32% *	Businesslike only	27	92	22%	20%	20%	44%	40%	32%	25%	27%	33%	23%	29%	27%	26%	27%
68%	Friendly too	73	247	78%	80%	80%	56%	60%	68%	75%	73%	67%	7.7%	71%	73%	74%	73%
			339	186	25	35	43	50	34	87	81	55	82	69	78	103	88
		100		55%	7%	10%	13%	15%	10%	26%	24%	16%	24%	20%	23%	30%	26%
								S									

Table 55

P		%	N	1	2	3	4	5	A	B	C	D	E	I	II	III	IV
	Q.66 Does your doctor look after all the people in your house?																
60%*	Yes	66	225	70	48%	69%	74%	52%	68%	75%	73%	69%	48%	84%	70%	64%	52%
28%	No	22	74	20%	12%	29%	16%	34%	26%	23%	26%	25%	12%	10%	22%	26%	26%
12%	Not applicable/respondent is single	12	41	10%	40%	3%	9%	14%	6%	2%	1%	6%	40%	6%	8%	10%	22%
0	Don't know	0	0	0	0	0	0	0	0	0	0	0	0	0	0	0	0
			340	187	25	35	43	50	34	88	81	55	82	69	78	103	89
		100		55%	7%	10%	13%	15%	10%	26%	24%	16%	24%	20%	23%	30%	26%
								HS					HS				HS
	Q.67 If yes: do you feel that you have a 'family doctor'?																
80%	Yes	82	185	86%	67%	79%	78%	77%	83%	89%	81%	71%	82%	78%	84%	82%	87%
12%	No	13	29	12%	8%	17%	19%	8%	9%	8%	19%	24%	5%	15%	11%	15%	9%
8%	Don't know	5	11	2%	25%	4%	3%	15%	9%	3%	0	5%	13%	7%	5%	3%	4%
			225	131	12	24	32	26	23	66	59	38	39	58	55	66	46
		100		58%	5%	11%	14%	12%	10%	29%	26%	17%	17%	26%	24%	29%	20%
								S					PS				
	Q.68 If yes: in general do you																
98%	Prefer a family doctor	98	181	97%	100%	100%	96%	100%	100%	93%	100%	100%	100%	96%	100%	100%	100%
1%	Don't know	2	3	2%	0	0	4%	0	0	5%	0	0	0	4%	2%	0	0
1%	Prefer different Drs.	1	1	1%	0	0	0	0	0	2%	0	0	0	0	2%	0	0
			185	113	8	19	25	20	19	59	48	27	32	45	46	54	40
		100		61%	4%	10%	14%	11%	10%	32%	26%	15%	17%	24%	25%	29%	22%

Table 56

P		%	N	1	2	3	4	5	A	B	C	D	E	I	II	III	IV
	Part 5 – The Doctor's method of work																
	Q.69 Do you feel your doctor is reluctant to visit you (or your children) at home?																
15%*	Yes	17	57	13%	4%	14%	40%	18%	29%	20%	17%	11%	11%	13%	19%	22%	11%
64%	No	64	219	64%	80%	71%	58%	60%	44%	56%	72%	73%	70%	61%	68%	59%	70%
4%	Sometimes	7	22	9%	4%	8%	2%	0	0	9%	4%	7%	8%	9%	5%	7%	6%
17%	Don't know	12	42	14%	12%	6%	0	22%	27%	15%	7%	9%	11%	17%	8%	12%	13%
			340	187	25	35	43	50	34	88	81	55	82	69	78	103	89
		100		55%	7%	10%	13%	15%	10%	26%	24%	16%	24%	20%	23%	30%	26%
								HS					PS				
	Q.70 If yes: do you ever feel your health has suffered as a result of this?																
7%	Yes	19	10	13%	100%	20%	33%	0	13%	17%	36%	20%	0	11%	15%	22%	25%
84%	No	74	39	83%	0	80%	53%	88%	62%	83%	50%	80%	100%	89%	77%	65%	75%
9%	Don't know	7	4	4%	0	0	13%	12%	25%	0	14%	0	0	0	8%	13%	0
			53	24	1	5	15	8	8	18	14	5	8	9	13	23	8
		100		45%	2%	9%	28%	15%	15%	34%	26%	9%	15%	17%	25%	43%	15%
	Q.71 Have you ever struggled to the surgery when you would have prefered the doctor to call?																
23%	Yes	24	75	20%		34%	33%	22%	12%	24%	29%	23%	25%	18%	22%	24%	30%
77%	No	76	239	80%		66%	65%	78%	85%	76%	71%	77%	75%	82%	78%	75%	70%
0	Don't know	0	1	0		0	2%	0	3%	0	0	0	0	0	0	1%	0
			315	187		35	43	50	34	88	80	52	61	65	74	95	81
		100		59%		11%	14%	16%	11%	28%	25%	17%	19%	21%	23%	30%	26%

Table 57

P		%	N	1	2 3	4	5	A	B	C	D	E	I	II	III	IV
Q.72 If yes: has your health ever suffered as a result of this?																
3%	Yes	9	7	3%	17%	29%	0	0	10%	14%	8%	7%	0	0	17%	13%
92%	No	84	62	89%	75%	64%	100%	75%	81%	86%	83%	87%	92%	94%	78%	78%
5%	Don't know	7	5	8%	8%	7%	0	25%	10%	0	8%	7%	8%	6%	4%	9%
			74	38	12	14	10	4	21	22	12	15	12	16	23	23
		100		51%	16%	19%	14%	5%	28%	30%	16%	20%	16%	22%	31%	31%
Q.73 Have you ever telephoned the doctor for advice?																
19%	Yes	27	85	31%	26%	35%	8%	24%	43%	35%	10%	10%	42%	26%	19%	26%
81%	No	73	228	69%	74%	65%	92%	76%	57%	65%	90%	88%	58%	73%	81%	74%
0	Don't know	0	1	1%	0	0	0	0	0	0	0	2%	0	1%	0	0
			314	186	35	43	50	33	88	80	52	61	65	74	96	81
		100		59%	11%	14%	16%	10%	28%	26%	17%	19%	21%	24%	30%	26%
												HS				PS
Q.74 Have you ever wanted to telephone the doctor for advice but did not do so?																
10%	Yes	12	39	15%	14%	9%	6%	3%	18%	11%	14%	10%	22%	12%	11%	7%
90%	No	87	273	84%	86%	91%	94%	97%	81%	89%	86%	88%	78%	85%	89%	93%
1%	Don't know	1	2	1%	0	0	0	0	1%	0	0	2%	0	3%	0	0
			314	186	35	43	50	33	88	80	52	61	65	74	94	81
		100		59%	11%	14%	16%	10%	28%	26%	17%	19%	21%	24%	30%	26%
																PS

Table 58

P		%	N	1	2	3	4	5	A	B	C	D	E	I	II	III	IV
	Part 6 – The use of para-medical staff																
	75–79: Apart from the doctors and the receptionists, do you know whether any of the following people work from the doctor's surgery?																
	Q75 Qualified nurses																
68%	Yes	78	245	79%		89%	91%	56%	50%	80%	88%	79%	77%	85%	81%	74%	74%
13%	No	9	28	9%		3%	5%	18%	18%	9%	1%	10%	13%	3%	10%	13%	9%
19%	Don't know	13	42	13%		9%	5%	26%	32%	11%	11%	11%	10%	12%	10%	14%	17%
			315	187		35	43	50	34	88	80	52	61	65	74	95	81
		100		59%		11%	14%	16%	11%	28%	25%	17%	19%	21%	23%	30%	26%
								S					S				
	Q76 Health visitors																
36%	Yes	47	148	48%		60%	56%	26%	32%	69%	56%	25%	30%	55%	55%	38%	43%
17%	No	14	43	13%		14%	7%	22%	21%	9%	6%	25%	16%	6%	16%	20%	12%
46%	Don't know	39	124	39%		26%	37%	52%	47%	22%	38%	50%	54%	39%	31%	42%	44%
			315	187		35	43	50	34	88	80	52	61	65	74	85	81
		100		59%		11%	14%	16%	11%	28%	25%	17%	19%	21%	23%	30%	26%
								PS					HS				
	Q77 Midwife																
36%	Yes	43	137	44%		43%	58%	30%	32%	67%	49%	25%	25%	49%	53%	39%	36%
20%	No	17	52	16%		26%	5%	22%	24%	11%	7%	33%	18%	6%	13%	21%	22%
44%	Don't know	40	126	40%		31%	37%	48%	44%	22%	44%	42%	57%	45%	34%	40%	42%
			315	187		35	43	50	34	88	80	52	61	65	74	95	81
		100		59%		11%	14%	16%	11%	28%	25%	17%	19%	21%	23%	30%	26%
													HS				

Table 59

P		%	N	1	2	3	4	5	A	B	C	D	E	I	II	III	IV
	Q.78 Social workers																
13%	Yes	13	41	13%		29%	0	12	6%	17%	14%	12%	12%	8%	18%	12%	15%
22%	No	22	70	23%		26%	16%	22%	35%	17%	17%	36%	16%	11%	24%	26%	25%
65%	Don't know	65	204	64%		46%	84%	66%	59%	66%	69%	52%	72%	81%	58%	62%	60%
			315	187		35	43	50	34	88	80	52	61	65	74	95	81
		100		59%		11%	14%	16%	11%	28%	25%	17%	19%	21%	23%	30%	26%
								S									
	Q.79 Marriage guidance counsellors																
5%	Yes	5	17	7%		3%	2%	4%	3%	7%	5%	8%	3%	6%	4%	6%	5%
28%	No	31	98	30%		50%	30%	24%	42%	31%	28%	40%	23%	20%	36%	35%	31%
67%	Don't know	63	199	63%		47%	67%	72%	55%	62%	67%	52%	74%	74%	60%	59%	64%
			314	187		34	43	50	33	88	80	52	61	65	74	95	80
		100		59%		11%	14%	16%	11%	28%	25%	17%	19%	21%	24%	30%	25%
	Q.80 Have you had any form of treatment from a nurse in the surgery after you had seen the doctor (e.g. having an injection, taking blood, syringing ears, checking your blood pressure)?																
36%	Yes	45	140	47%		51%	53%	26%	27%	50%	45%	44%	47%	46%	49%	44%	41%
64%	No	55	173	53%		49%	47%	74%	73%	50%	55%	56%	53%	54%	51%	56%	59%
0	Don't know	0	0	0		0	0	0	0	0	0	0	0	0	0	0	0
			313	185		35	43	50	33	88	80	52	60	65	74	94	80
		100		59%		11%	14%	16%	10%	28%	26%	17%	19%	21%	24%	30%	26%
								PS									

Table 60

P		%	N	1	2	3	4	5	A	B	C	D	E	I	II	III	IV
	Q.81 If yes: would you have preferred the doctor to have done that for you?																
6%	Yes	6	8	4%		6%	13%	8%	0	7%	14%	0	0	3%	3%	7%	9%
93%	No	93	130	94%		94%	87%	92%	89%	91%	86%	100%	100%	97%	97%	88%	91%
1%	Don't know	1	2	2%		0	0	0	11%	2%	0	0	0	0	0	5%	0
			140	86		18	23	13	9	44	36	33	28	30	36	41	33
		100		61%		13%	16%	9%	6%	31%	26	16%	20%	21%	26%	29%	24%
													PS				
	Q.82 Do you think that nurses should work in the surgery doing that sort of job for the doctor?																
94%	Yes	93	292	95%		86%	93%	94%	100%	94%	91%	94%	90%	97%	92%	93%	92%
4%	No	4	12	3%		9%	2%	4%	0	5%	8%	2%	2%	0	5%	2%	8%
2%	Don't know	3	9	2%		6%	5%	2%	0	1%	1%	4%	8%	3%	3%	5%	0
			313	185		35	43	50	34	88	80	51	60	65	74	94	80
		100		59%		11%	14%	16%	11%	28%	26%	16%	19%	21%	24%	30%	26%
	Q.83 If you (or your children) had a minor complaint (e.g. a septic skin, a rash, earache) and the nurse treated this instead of the doctor, would you mind?																
14%	Yes	19	5	18%		31%	21%	8%	12%	17%	21%	23%	16%	15%	22%	14%	24%
80%	No	76	241	77%		69%	72%	84%	79%	80%	73%	73%	80%	77%	72%	83%	74%
6%	Sometimes	4	13	4%		0	5%	8%	9%	2%	6%	2%	3%	8%	7%	2%	1%
0	Don't know	1	2	1%		0	2%	0	0	1%	0	2%	0	0	0	1%	1%
			314	186		35	43	50	34	88	80	51	61	65	74	94	81
		100		59%		11%	14%	16%	11%	28%	26%	16%	19%	21%	24%	30%	26%

Table 61

P		%	N	1	2	3	4	5	A	B	C	D	E	I	II	III	IV
	Q.84 Has a nurse ever visited you (or your children) at home when in fact you had sent for the doctor?																
10%	Yes	22	68	5%		31%	100%	8%	12%	30%	25%	10%	21%	16%	15%	32%	21%
90%	No	78	245	94%		69%	0	92%	85%	70%	75%	90%	79%	84%	84%	68%	79%
0	Don't know	0	1	1%		0	0	0	3%	0	0	0	0	0	1%	0	0
			314	186		35	43	50	34	87	80	52	61	64	74	95	81
		100		59%		11%	14%	16%	11%	28%	25%	17%	19%	20%	24%	30%	26%
	If No, skip to Q.88							HS					PS				
	Q.85 If yes: was the advice and treatment satisfactory?																
77%	Yes	74	51	70%		73%	74%	80%	75%	81%	52%	80%	92%	70%	75%	67%	88%
22%	No	25	17	30%		27%	23%	20%	25%	15%	48%	20%	8%	30%	17%	33%	12%
0	Don't know	1	1	0		0	2%	0	0	4%	0	0	0	0	8%	0	0
			69	10		11	43	5	4	26	21	5	13	10	12	30	17
		100		15%		16%	62%	7%	6%	38%	30%	7%	19%	14%	17%	44%	25%
	Q.86 Do you think your health, or your children's health, suffered because the nurse came rather than the doctor?																
11%	Yes	18	12	20%		20%	19%	0	0	8%	37%	20%	15%	20%	27%	17%	12%
88%	No	79	53	80%		80%	77%	100%	100%	88%	58%	80%	85%	80%	64%	80%	88%
1%	Don't know	3	2	0		0	5%	0	0	4%	5%	0	0	0	9%	3%	0
			67	10		10	43	4	4	26	19	5	13	10	11	29	17
		100		15%		15%	64%	6%	6%	39%	28%	8%	19%	15%	16%	43%	25%
	Q.87 Would you have preferred the doctor?																
46%	Yes	55	37	70%		60%	54%	25%	25%	50%	58%	60%	69%	70%	73%	45%	53%
54%	No	43	29	30%		40%	44%	75%	75%	46%	42%	40%	31%	30%	27%	52%	47%
1%	Don't know	2	1	0		0	2%	0	0	4%	0	0	0	0	0	3%	0
			67	10		10	43	4	4	26	19	5	13	10	11	29	17
		100		15%		15%	64%	6%	6%	39%	28%	8%	19%	15%	16%	43%	25%
	Skip to Question 90																

Table 62

P		%	N	1	2	3	4	5	A	B	C	D	E	I	II	III	IV
Q.88	If the nurse came when you had sent for the doctor would you mind?																
39%	Yes	40	99	41%		42%	0	38%	48%	34%	42%	47%	35%	41%	38%	43%	40%
46%	No	46	112	45%		50%	0	47%	48%	46%	37%	47%	53%	41%	44%	48%	49%
13%	Sometimes	12	30	12%		8%	0	13%	3%	18%	17%	4%	12%	17%	16%	9%	8%
2%	Don't know	2	4	2%		0	0	2%	0	2%	3%	2%	0	2%	2%	0	3%
			245	176		24	0	45	29	61	59	47	49	54	61	65	65
		100		72%		10%		18%	12%	25%	24%	19%	20%	22%	25%	27%	27%
Q.89	Do you feel that this would be a satisfactory system of care?																
36%	Yes	38	92	36%		54%	0	34%	45%	31%	31%	36%	51%	31%	33%	43%	46%
41%	No	44	109	47%		42%	0	36%	48%	49%	42%	49%	35%	44%	46%	42%	46%
23%	Sometimes	17	41	15%		4%	0	30%	7%	20%	25%	13%	12%	20%	21%	15%	11%
1%	Don't know	1	3	2%		0	0	0	0	0	2%	2%	2%	4%	0	0	2%
			245	177		24	0	44	29	61	59	47	49	54	61	65	65
		100		72%		10%		18%	12%	25%	24%	19%	20%	22%	25%	27%	27%
Q.90	Has a nurse ever visited you or your children at home as a follow-up from the doctor's visit?																
22%*	Yes	33	112	24%	96%	56%	42%	12%	12%	34%	33%	27%	45%	28%	25%	42%	34%
78	No	67	225	76%	0	44%	58%	88%	88%	66%	67%	73%	54%	72%	75%	58%	65%
0	Don't know	0	1	0	4%	0	0	0	0	0	0	0	1%	0	0	0	1%
			338	187	25	34	43	49	34	88	79	55	82	69	77	102	89
		100		55%	7%	10%	13%	15%	10%	26%	23%	16%	24%	20%	23%	30%	26%
								HS					PS				

If No, or Don't know skip to Q.96

Table 63

P		%	N	1	2	3	4	5	A	B	C	D	E	I	II	III	IV
Q.91	Was the advice and treatment satisfactory?																
95%*	Yes	94	105	93%	92%	100%	89%	100%	75%	100%	92%	87%	95%	100%	95%	88%	97%
4%	No	4	4	7%	0	0	6%	0	0	0	8%	7%	3%	0	5%	5%	3%
1%	Don't know	3	3	0	8%	0	6%	0	25%	0	0	7%	3%	0	0	7%	0
			112	45	24	19	18	6	4	30	26	15	37	19	19	43	30
		100		40%	21%	17%	16%	5%	4%	27%	23%	13%	33%	17%	17%	38%	27%
													PS				
Q.92	Did you feel confident that the nurse would report any new problems back to the doctor?																
94%*	Yes	93	104	93%	96%	95%	83%	100%	50%	93%	96%	93%	95%	100%	89%	88%	97%
4%	No	3	3	7%	0	0	0	0	0	3%	4%	7%	0	0	5%	5%	0
2%	Don't know	4	5	0	4%	5%	17%	0	50%	3%	0	0	5%	0	5%	7%	3%
			112	45	24	19	18	6	4	30	26	15	37	19	19	43	30
		100		40%	21%	17%	16%	5%	4%	27%	23%	13%	33%	17%	17%	38%	27%
													HS				
Q.93	If Yes: Did you feel confident that the doctor would take the necessary action?																
100% *	Yes	100	104	100%	100%	100%	100%	100%	100%	100%	100%	100%	100%	100%	100%	100%	100%
	·		104	42	23	18	15	6	2	28	25	14	35	19	17	38	29
		100%		40%	22%	17%	14%	6%	2%	27%	24%	13%	34%	18%	16%	37%	28%
Q.94	Do you think your health suffered as a result of the nurse's visit?																
0 *	Yes	2	2	0	0	0	11%	0	25%	0	4%	0	0	0	0	5%	0
99%	No	97	109	100%	96%	100%	89%	100%	75%	100%	96%	100%	97%	100%	100%	95%	97%
1%	Don't know	1	1	0	4%	0	0	0	0	0	0	0	3%	0	0	0	3%
			112	45	24	19	18	6	4	30	26	15	37	19	19	43	30
		100		40%	21%	17%	14%	5%	4%	27%	23%	13%	33%	17%	17%	38%	27%

Table 64

P		%	N	1	2	3	4	5	A	B	C	D	E	I	II	III	IV
Q.95	Would you have preferred the doctor?																
27%*	Yes	26	29	18%	38%	37%	17%	33%	25%	23%	23%	27%	30%	11%	26%	35%	27%
66%	No	71	79	78%	62%	63%	78%	50%	75%	73%	69%	73%	68%	84%	74%	63%	73%
6%	Sometimes	3	3	2%	0	0	6%	17%	0	0	8%	0	3%	0	0	2%	0
1%	Don't know	1	1	2%	0	0	0	0	0	3%	0	0	0	5%	0	0	0
			112	45	24	19	18	6	4	30	26	15	37	19	19	43	30
		100		40%	21%	17%	16%	5%	4%	27%	23%	13%	33%	17%	17%	38%	27%
	Skip to Q.100																
Q.96	If the nurse came to follow up your illness after the doctor had seen you initially, would you mind?																
4%	Yes	4	9	3%	0	6%	8%	5%	7%	3%	4%	3%	4%	0	7%	5%	3%
93%	No	92	210	94%	100%	94%	80%	93%	93%	95%	89%	92%	91%	94%	90%	92%	93%
3%	Sometimes	4	9	3%	0	0	12%	2%	0	2%	7%	5%	4%	6%	3%	3%	3%
0	Don't know	0	0	0	0	0	0	0	0	0	0	0	0	0	0	0	0
			228	142	1	16	25	44	30	59	55	40	44	51	59	60	58
		100		62%	0	7%	11%	19%	13%	26%	24%	18%	19%	22%	26%	26%	25%
Q.97	Would you feel confident that the nurse would report any new problems you may have back to the doctor?																
92%	Yes	91	207	89%	0	88%	100%	93%	93%	95%	91%	87%	86%	90%	91%	97%	85%
1%	No	2	4	2%	0	6%	0	0	0	0	2%	5%	2%	0	2%	0	5%
8%	Don't know	7	17	9%	100%	6%	0	7%	7%	5%	7%	8%	11%	10%	7%	3%	10%
			228	142	1	16	25	44	30	59	55	40	44	51	59	60	58
		100		62%	0	7%	11%	19%	13%	26%	24%	18%	19%	22%	26%	26%	25%

PS

Table 65

P		%	N	1	2	3	4	5	A	B	C	D	E	I	II	III	IV
Q.98	If Yes: would you feel confident that the doctor would take the necessary action?																
93%	Yes	95	196	95%		86%	100%	93%	100%	95%	92%	94%	95%	96%	96%	93%	94%
3%	No	3	6	1%		14%	0	8%	0	4%	6%	3%	0	2%	4%	3%	2%
4%	Don't know	2	5	4%		0	0	0	0	2%	2%	3%	5%	2%	0	3%	4%
			207	128		14	25	40	28	56	50	35	38	46	54	58	49
		100		62%		7%	12%	19%	14%	27%	24%	17%	18%	22%	26%	28%	24%
								PS									
Q.99	Do you feel that this would be a satisfactory system of care?																
86%	Yes	86	195	86%	100%	87%	84%	88%	93%	86	83%	82%	89%	86%	79%	93%	86%
7%	No	8	18	8%	0	13%	8%	5%	3%	9%	11%	8%	7%	10%	14%	2%	7%
7%	Don't know	6	13	6%	0	0	8%	7%	3%	5%	6%	10%	4%	4%	7%	5%	7%
			226	142	1	15	25	43	30	59	53	40	44	51	58	59	58
		100		63%	0	7%	11%	19%	13%	26%	23%	18%	20%	23%	26%	26%	26%
Q.100	Have you ever used the health visitor's services?																
14% *	Yes	18	61	18%	12%	21%	28%	10%	6%	40%	22%	6%	5%	19%	20%	13%	23%
86%	No	81	273	82%	76%	79%	70%	90%	94%	59%	78%	94%	91%	80%	79%	87%	75%
0	Don't know	1	4	0	12%	0	2%	0	0	1%	0	0	4%	1%	1%	0	2%
			338	187	25	34	43	49	34	88	79	55	82	69	77	102	89
		100		55%	7%	10%	13%	15%	10%	26%	23%	16%	24%	20%	23%	30%	26%
								HS					HS				
Q.101	Do you feel it is a good idea for the health visitor to work on the same premises as the doctor?																
78%*	Yes	75	253	81%	17%	85%	70%	78%	56%	88%	87%	78%	56%	84%	77%	70%	74%
4%	No	3	10	2%	4%	0	5%	6%	18%	1%	1%	0	2%	1%	4%	4%	2%
18%	Don't know	22	74	17%	79%	15%	26%	16%	26%	11%	11%	22%	42%	15%	19%	26%	24%
			337	187	24	34	43	49	34	88	79	55	81	69	77	102	88
		100		55%	7%	10%	13%	15%	10%	26%	23%	16%	24%	20%	23%	30%	26%
								HS					HS				

Table 66

Q 102 Do you have any children?
- Yes
- No

Q 103 Are any of them under the age of seven?
- Yes
- No

(Questions 104-118 are to be asked only of women with children under the age of seven. Everyone else skip to question 119)

Q 104 Have you attended the surgery during the last three years for ante-natal care during pregnancy?
- Yes
- No
- Don't know

If No skip to question 108

Table 67

Q 105 If yes: were you ever seen by the midwife without seeing the doctor?

- Yes
- No
- Don't know

Q 106 If yes: did you feel the midwife did the same job as the doctor?

- Yes
- No
- Don't know

Q 107 If the midwife provided the routine ante-natal care with the doctor seeing you only occasionally or if things were not normal, would you be

- Very happy
- Happy
- No opinion
- Unhappy
- Very unhappy

Table 68

Q 108	Have you attended the surgery well-baby clinic?	
		Yes
		No
		Don't know
Q 109	If yes: did you attend regularly?	
		Yes
		No
		Don't know
Q 110	Was the clinic	
		Well organised
		Organised
		No opinion/don't know
		Unorganised
		Very unorganised

Table 69

Q 111 When you attended the well-baby clinic did you find that the advice which you received from the health visitor was

Very unhelpful
Unhelpful
No opinion/don't know
Helpful
Very helpful

(asked of mothers who have attended immunisation sessions)

Q112 Did you find that the immunisation sessions run by the health visitor were

Very helpful
Helpful
No opinion/don't know
Unhelpful
Very unhelpful

Q 113 Has the health visitor ever given you advice about you or your children's problems (e.g. bedwetting in children)

Yes
No
Don't know

Table 70

Q 114 If yes: Did you find this to be

- Very acceptable
- Acceptable
- No opinion/don't know
- Unacceptable
- Very unacceptable

Q 115 Have or would you ever seek advice from the health visitor about your children when they were not well?

- Yes
- No
- Sometimes
- Don't know

Q 116 If yes: was or would this be

- Very unacceptable
- Unacceptable
- No opinion/don't know
- Acceptable
- Very acceptable

Table 71

Q 117	Have you ever received advice about your children's health from a qualified nurse?	
		Yes
		No
		Don't know
Q 118	Did or would you mind?	
		Yes
		No
		Don't know
Q 119	Do you ever get repeat prescriptions without seeing the doctor?	
		Yes
		No
		Don't know
Q 120	If yes: is this system satisfactory?	
		Yes
		No
		Don't know

Table 72

Q 121 How do you get your doctor after midnight in an emergency?

- Ring surgery
- Ring doctor's home
- Call at the surgery
- Call at doctor's home
- Ring 999
- Ring police
- Other
- Don't know

The following five questions were asked of chronic housebound patients only

Q 122 Does the nurse call to see you from time to time in place of the doctor?

- Yes
- No
- Don't know

Q 123 If yes: on these occasions, do you feel that the doctor and the nurse both do the same job when they see you?

- Yes
- No
- Don't know

Table 73

Q 124 Do you ever feel your health has suffered as a result of the nurse visiting you on these occasions rather than the doctor?

- Yes
- No
- Don't know

Q 125 Do you feel confident that the nurse will report any new problems you may have back to the doctor?

- Yes
- No
- Don't know

Q 126 If yes: do you feel confident that the doctor will take the necessary action?

- Yes
- No
- Don't know

INDEX

Administrative secretaries, 48, 49
Allen, W.H., 40
Ambler, M., 40
Anaemia, 59
Ante-natal care, 29, 39, 40; by midwives, 65, 127-8
Appointments system, 17, 27-8, 62, 122-3, 131-2
Association of Medical Secretaries, 17
Attachment of Nursing Services to General Practice, Joint Working Party on, 17-18, 34-5, 37
Attendance, *see* Surgery attendance

BMA Planning Unit report (1970), 13
Bebbington, R. 29
Bevan, J.M., 137
Binnie, G.A.C., 26
Briggs Report (1972), 38
Buckoke, Y.E., 35, 40

Cartwright, A., 13, 29, 30, 135, 136-7
Certificate of incapacity to work, 124, 133, 161
Cervical smear tests, 48
Childbirth, 41
Children, 59
Chronic illness, 36, 58, 63, 112, 118, 128
Clergy, 48, 49
Clinical Nursing Studies, Joint Board of, 38
Consultants, 62
Consultations, 24-31, 55-60; and geographical area, 25-8; and proportion of patients, 99; by age group, 89; by disease, 81-3; by nurses, 106; by team, 107; follow up rates, 28, 59, 62; initiated by patients and by doctors, 97-8; length of, 132; non-consulters, 102-3; number per patient, 86; satisfaction with, 158-62; variations in rate of, 31, 58-9, 104-5
Cunningham, D.J., 137

Data collection (survey), 68-72
Dawson report (1920), 13
Department of Health and Social Security, 16, 21, 31, 36, 42
Diagnosis: most frequent, by consultation, 82; multiple, 83; referrals, 62, 84-5
Diagnostic tests, 54, 63
Disease: analysis of consultations by, 81-4; prevalence, 53-4
Distance from surgery, 25-6, 120
Doctors: age of, 28-9; attitudes towards patients, 28; changing, 51; communication with patients, 131; concern for patients, 124-5, 112; difficulty in seeing, 123; number in group practice, 14; own doctor system, 50-1, 62-3, 123-5; schedules, 50-1, 52; *see also* Norton practice
Donaldson, R.J., 20

Eimerl, T.S., 31
Elderly, care of, 39, 59

Family Doctor's Charter, 13, 137
Family planning, 48
Family Practitioner Committee, 16
Forman, J.A.S., 38, 42
Fry, J., 20, 25, 29, 40

General Medical Services, Joint Working Party on (1973), 136
General practice, 13-23
General Practice Finance Corporation, 15
Gillie Report (1963), 13, 18
Gilmore, M., 35
Group practice, 8; allowance, 15; centres, 14-15; trend towards, 13-14; *see also* Norton Practice

Hasler, J.C., 18, 36, 38
Health Centres – a Design Guide (DHSS), 14
Health service objectives, 137-8
Health visitors, 19-21, 39-40, 48, 71, 117, 166; satisfaction with, 127-8; workload, 59-60, 64
Hockey, L., 34
Hodes, C., 38

Hodgkin, K., 29
Home visit cards, 77
Home visits, 25-31 *passim,* 37, 55-66 *passim,* 125-6; by age group 91; made by nurses, 35, 59; and proportion of patients, 101
Hopkins, E.J., 26, 29
Hospitals, 51-2, 78; admissions, 85; casualty departments, 49; obstetric facilities, 51; referrals to, 53-4, 62, 84-5
Households, contact with, 88
Howard, A.L., 19

Immunisation schemes, 39, 40, 50, 128, 177
Industrial medical centres, 49
Infant care, 39-40, 48, 128, 176-7
Influenza, 31
Integrated Health Services, Report on, 34, 37
Intensive care, 53-4, 113
Irvine, D., 15, 16, 19, 20

Jefferys, M., 41

Kedward, H.N., 30
Kuenssberg, E.V., 36-7

Laboratory tests, 51
Lance, H., 26
List, size of, 26, 27, 62, 66; determination of, 68
Local authority health centres, 14-15
Logan, W.P.D., 24, 25
Longmore, H.J.A., 26

McKnight, S.G., 31
Manning, A.D., 31
Manpower shortages, 136
Marriage guidance counsellors, 39, 48, 49, 167
Marsh, G.N., 24-5, 26, 28, 30, 31, 36, 53
Medical Secretaries Handbook, 17
Midwives, 21, 40-41, 117, 166; ante-natal care by, 65; satisfaction with, 127-8
Miners, 25, 29
Minor injuries, 59
Moore, M.S., 37
Morrell, D.C., 26, 28, 29, 30, 31, 68

Non-medical problems, 159
Normal users, 113-114
Norton practice, 46-52; appointment system, 122-3, 131-2, 152-5; criticisms of, 125; doctor's method of working, 125-7; hospital services, 51-2; nurses, 126-7, 149-51; own doctor system, 123-5, 156-8; patients, 46-7; patients' satisfaction with their care, 119-28, 158-62; premises, 47-8, 119, 120, 143-5; receptionists, 120-2, 146-8; staff, 47-9; working methods, 49-51
Nurse-first users, 113
Nurses, 9, 17-19; 34-8; attitudes to, 121, 126-7; at the Norton practice, 48, 166; consultations by, 106; follow up visits by, 127; local authority, 71; number required, 18; satisfaction with treatment by, 126-7, 130, 167-72; training, 17, 64, 130; workload, 59; *see also* state registered nurses *and* state enrolled nurses

Obstetric care, 21, 29, 51, 71

Patient satisfaction survey, 111-39; findings, 119-28; interview, 114-17; questionnaire, 111-12, 116-17; respondents, 117-18; role of surveys, 135-9; sample, 113-14, 118; validity of findings, 133-4
Patients: age of 28-9, 46; attendances, 86, 90, 93; causing heaviest work load, 57-8; characteristics of, 55-6; communication with health care team, 131; computerised information storage on, 69; distance from surgery, 25-6, 47; expectations, 135-6; female, 55; mobility of, 47, 56, 95; newly arrived, 30-31, 47; number of consultations, 86; satisfaction with care received, 61-6, 109-39; sex of, 46; social class of, 46-7, 93, 94, 103; visits to, 87, 91, 92, 93, 94, 96
Patients' Association, 136
Personal doctor system, 50-1, 62-3, 123-5
Picken, B., 30
Posner, B.H., 25, 31
Post-natal care, 40-1
Practice Nurse, The, 36
Pregnancy *see* ante-natal care
Prescriptions, 124, 161

Primary health care team, 15-16, 34-43; *see also specific members of team*
Primary Health Care Teams, 35, 38, 42
Psychiatric illness, 61-2

Ratoff, L., 42
Receptionists, 48, 120-2
Record system, 50; card, 73-4
Respiratory infections, 53, 59
Richardson, I.M., 28
Rowland, A.J., 37
Royal College of General Practitioners, 24, 36
Royal College of General Practitioners, *North West Merseyside Survey,* 17, 18, 20
Royal Commission on Medical Education, 13
Rural areas, 25-6, 27

Scot, R., 30
Secretarial staff, 16-17, 48, 120-2
Seebohm Report (1968), 41
Single handed practice, 8, 13
Social class, 29-30, 56, 60; and consultations, 92, 98; and home visits, 93, 94; and household contact, 94; and surgery attendances, 93, 94; and the survey analysis, 69-70; effect on workload, 65
Social Work Support for the Health Services, 42
Social workers, 39, 41-3, 48, 49, 166
Standing Medical Advisory Committee, 18, 21, 35, 37
Standing Nursing Advisory Committee, 35
State enrolled nurses, 34, 38, 39, 48
State registered nurses, 34, 37-8, 39, 48, 63-4
Surgery attendance, 86; analysis by age group, 90; and proportion of patients, 100; cards, 76; difficulty with, 120
Surgery attendance/home visit ratio, 25, 29, 55, 61; analysis is by age totals, 92; analysis by social class, 94; analysis by time on list, 96

Taylor, S., 13
Trainee practitioners, 14, 48

Urban areas, 25-6

Wamoscher, Z., 29, 31
Warin, J.F., 18, 20, 21, 34, 40
Weston Smith, J., 18, 35
Williams, W.O., 24, 25, 27, 28-9
Wolfe, S., 42
Women doctors, 124, 158
Workloads, 55-66; doctors', 24-31,36, 56-7; factors affecting, 61-2; health visitor's, 59-60; midwife's, 60; nurse's, 59; social worker's, 60; statistics of, 81-107; *see also* consultations
Wright, 24-5, 27, 28-9, 31

X-rays, 51-2

For Product Safety Concerns and Information please contact our EU representative GPSR@taylorandfrancis.com Taylor & Francis Verlag GmbH, Kaufingerstraße 24, 80331 München, Germany